Childhood Cancer Management

Childhood Cancer Management

A PRACTICAL HANDBOOK

C.R. Pinkerton MD, FRCPI
Consultant Paediatric Oncologist
Royal Marsden Hospital
Surrey, UK

P. Cushing RGN, RSCN, Onc Cert
Senior Sister
Royal Marsden Hospital
Surrey, UK

and

B. Sepion RGN, RSCN, Onc Cert, FETC
Clinical Teacher and Clinical Nurse Specialist
Royal Marsden Hospital
Surrey, UK

CHAPMAN & HALL MEDICAL
London · Glasgow · New York · Tokyo · Melbourne · Madras

Published by Chapman & Hall, 2–6 Boundary Row, London SE1 8HN

Chapman & Hall, 2–6 Boundary Row, London SE1 8HN, UK

Blackie Academic & Professional, Wester Cleddens Road, Bishopbriggs, Glasgow G64 2NZ, UK

Chapman & Hall Inc., One Penn Plaza, 41st Floor, New York NY10119, USA

Chapman & Hall Japan, Thomson Publishing Japan, Hirakawacho Nemoto Building, 6F, 1-7-11 Hirakawa-cho, Chiyoda-ku, Tokyo 102, Japan

Chapman & Hall Australia, Thomas Nelson Australia, 102 Dodds Street, South Melbourne, Victoria 3205, Australia

Chapman & Hall India, R. Seshadri, 32 Second Main Road, CIT East, Madras 600 035, India

First edition 1994

© 1994 C.R. Pinkerton, P. Cushing and B. Sepion

Typeset in 10/12 Times by Best-set Typesetter Ltd., Hong Kong.
Printed in Great Britain by the Alden Press Ltd., Oxford

ISBN 0 412 41080 X

A catalogue record for this book is available from the British Library

Library of Congress Cataloging-in-Publication data available

∞ Printed on permanent acid-free text paper, manufactured in accordance with the proposed ANSI/NISO Z 39.48-199X and ANSI Z 39.48-1984

Contents

Acknowledgements

We are grateful to the nursing, medical and pharmacy staff on the children's ward of the Royal Marsden for their helpful suggestions, and to Joan Malings for invaluable assistance with the manuscript.

Impact of diagnosis on the family

Cancer is the most feared of diseases and the public generally have an unrealistic and negative attitude towards it. Many are over-pessimistic about its treatment and outcome and despite education to improve public awareness about prevention, treatment and improved cure rates, it is still seen as a 'death threat' (Patterson and Aitken-Swan, 1954; Briggs and Wakefield, 1967; Hobbs, 1967; Williams, Cruikshank and Walker, 1972).

A belief in the value of early detection (often unfounded) may explain the anger and increased anxiety of parents who feel signs and symptoms were not investigated quickly or thoroughly enough. Delay in diagnosis is not uncommon; general practitioners/paediatricians in district general hospitals may only see one or two cases of childhood cancer, the signs and symptoms of which can be similar to many other childhood illnesses. Parents will require help to re-establish trusting relationships with these professionals who may be asked to participate in the child's care following the commencement of treatment.

Most children with a suspected malignancy will now be referred to a regional centre for paediatric oncology. This is in the child's best interest as there is access to the most up to date therapy (Nicholson, 1990). The chance of survival with least sequelae is also better (Stiller, 1988).

Once cancer is suspected there is intense medical activity and it is likely to become a period of extreme stress and anxiety. It has been shown that at this time to some parents the suspicion of cancer is worse than the confirmation; to others, however, a paediatric illness with a worse prognosis, e.g. cystic fibrosis may seem preferable (Barbor, 1983).

The child and family are surrounded by unfamiliar faces in an unfamiliar environment with the fear of the diagnosis of cancer and all the stresses that this arouses. Stress is a complex range of physiological and psychological responses; parents may experience feelings of fear, guilt, anxiety, tension, anger, hopelessness and depression. They need the opportunity to recognize that these feelings are not abnormal and may require 'permission' or the provision of appropriate facilities to express them, e.g. privacy to cry or open spaces to scream and shout. Health care professionals caring for children with cancer have recognized the complexity of providing care for the child and family. No one health professional can completely meet a family's needs and a multidisciplinary approach is more likely to be able to provide comprehensive care that supports the family through the disease and its treatment (Herch and Wiener, 1989). Effective communication is vital in all aspects of patient and family care (Watson, 1983). Initially, as trusting relationships are being established, non-verbal communication, using eye contact, touch and listening skills are very effective.

The value of information given on admission to hospital must be emphasized (Elms and Leonard, 1966). Explanations prior to diagnostic tests and surgical procedures (Hayward, 1975; Boore, 1978) all reduce anxiety, pain and side effects in the majority of patients. Complete information concerning the hospital, staff, routines and commonly used language may need to be given repeatedly in order for it to be fully understood. It is preferable, therefore, that whenever possible information packs about the ward − providing details about the ward layout, routine, facilities for parents and advice on what to bring into hospital − are sent prior to admission or are available on admission. Being expected and greeted by name also helps families to feel welcome.

On admission a calm and reassuring atmosphere is conducive to lowering the parents' and child's anxieties. Observation for acute medical conditions that may require immediate intervention should be carried out by a skilled practitioner. Providing time for the child and family to become acclimatised to their new environment may also help to reduce their stress and anxiety. Relief of symptoms such as pain should be seen as a priority. Providing effective pain control encourages the establishment of a trusting relationship between nurse and patient and the nurse and family (Smith, 1976).

It has been reported that 60% of children with cancer experience pain due to disease or procedures (Miser et al., 1987). Patients who are experiencing pain may find it very difficult to cope and co-operate with admission procedures and diagnostic tests. Only once it has been established that the patient is in a stable and comfortable condition can time be spent sharing information that will assist the family and patient through the admission procedure and diagnostic tests.

The confirmation of diagnosis may not be a medical emergency but it almost certainly will be an emotional one (Barbor, 1983). One dilemma is whether to rush ahead with diagnostic procedures in order to confirm the diagnosis and therefore give the child and family details of prognosis, treatment plans and goals or to give them time to settle in, establish trusting relationships and adequately prepare for the often numerous investigative procedures.

The improvement in the treatment and cure of childhood cancers is dependent on intensive and rigorous investigation and staging procedures. To help the child and family prepare for and comply with these procedures the health care professionals must have knowledge about the number and type of investigative procedures that each diagnosis requires. The knowledge must include the implications to the child, e.g. is it painful, invasive or requires the patient to co-operate by laying still, holding their breath or being separated from their carer. To assist in preparing the child information including their previous experiences with hospital – if any – their ability to cope with unfamiliar and threatening procedures, their level of development, their coping mechanisms/ strategies and understanding of the reason for hospitalization will be useful. The parents possess this type of knowledge, but it must be remembered that the parents' anxiety and stress levels may prevent them or inhibit them from participating in planning their child's care at that stage.

Considerable adaptation to changed circumstances may be required. It has been reported that parents of a child with a chronic illness when confronted with the task of parenting a child who is considered less than perfect may initially have to grieve for the loss of their once healthy child (Austin, 1990). Being able to participate in the patient's care and being part of the caring team are factors that help families cope when facing the diagnosis of cancer (Martocchio, 1985).

What to tell a child who has a life-threatening disease is an issue that has only recently been addressed. The general agreement now is that children, following careful assessment of their level of development, chronological age and family situation, should be given appropriately detailed information about their disease, its treatment and prognosis (Spinetta, Rigler and Karon, 1973; Eisler, 1984).

Certainly if children are to co-operate with painful, uncomfortable, threatening procedures or procedures that inflict restrictions on their activities of daily living, e.g. observing a fast prior to an anaesthetic, they must have an understanding of why. Children can demonstrate their ability to remain brave for one-off procedures but for the child facing the diagnosis of cancer, investigations and staging procedures occur with regularity throughout the treatment. Diagnostic tests should not be so frightening or painful that the child is then frightened of the treatment. It is important, therefore, to establish a means of gaining the patient's trust and co-operation to comply with the procedures and subsequent treatment.

Play therapist/specialists have an important role in facilitating and assessing a child's coping abilities and strategies. Structured play helps to prepare patients for different procedures and gives opportunities to act out fears, misconceptions, anxieties and other emotions. The play may include observing the procedure being carried out on a doll and then encouraging the child to be the doctor/nurse. Some children may find it helpful to observe another child undergoing the procedure and discussing how the other child 'coped'.

Practising or having a rehearsal may also be useful to some patients — others may prefer just to 'get on with it'. Some patients may cope by having 'goals' or positive reinforcers. However, bribes in the form of presents should be avoided as children can quickly learn the philosophy of 'the louder I cry the bigger the present' — which does not help the child to cope and can create many difficulties for the whole family in the future. Parental involvement — helping the child and parent establish their roles is very important prior to the procedure (Patterson, 1988).

REFERENCES

Austin, J. (1990) Assessment of coping mechanisms used by parents and children with chronic illness. *American Journal of Maternal and Child Nursing*, **15**, 98–102.

Barbor, P. (1983) Emotional aspects of malignant disease in children. *Maternal and Child Health*, **8**, 320–327.

Boore, J. (1978) *A Prescription for Recovery*. Royal College of Nursing, London.

Briggs, J.E. and Wakefield, J. (1967) Public opinion on cancer, a survey of knowledge among women in Lancaster. Department of Social Research, Christie Hospital and Holt Radium Institute, Manchester.

Eisler, C. (1984) Communicating with sick children. *Journal of Child Psychology and Psychiatry*, **25**, 181–189.

Elms, R. and Leonard, R. (1966) Effects of nursing approaches during admission. *Nursing Research*, **15**, 39–48.

Hayward, J. (1975) Information. A prescription against pain. Royal College of Nursing, London.

Hersh, S.P. and Wiener, L.S. (1989) Psychosocial support for the family of the child with cancer, in *Principles and Practice of Paediatric Oncology* (eds P.A. Pizzo and D.G. Poplack) **42**, 897–913.

Hobbs, P. (1967) Public opinion of cancer – a survey of knowledge and attitudes among women on Merseyside. Merseyside Cancer Education Committee, Liverpool.

Martocchio, B. (1985) Family coping – helping families to help themselves. *Seminars in Oncology Nursing*, **1**(4), 292–297.

Miser, A.W., Dothage, J.A. and Wesley, R.A. (1987) The prevalence of pain in a paediatric and young adult cancer population. *Pain*, **29**, 73–83.

Nicholson, A. (1990) Childhood cancer – an overview, in *The Child with Cancer – Nursing Care* (ed. J. Thompson), Ch. 1, Scutari, London.

Patterson, J.M. (1988) Chronic illness in children and the impact on families, in

Chronic Disability (ed. C.S. Chilman), C.A. Sage Publications Inc., Newbury Park, pp. 69–107.

Patterson, R. and Aitken-Swan, J. (1954) Public opinion on cancer – a survey among women in the Manchester area. *Lancet*, **ii**, 857–861.

Smith, M. (1976) The pre-schooler and pain, in *Current Practice in Paediatric Nursing* (eds P. Brandt, P. Chinn and M. Smith), C.V. Mosby, St Louis.

Spinetta, J.J., Rigler, D. and Karon, M. (1973) Anxiety and the dying child. *Paediatrics*, **52**, 841–845.

Stiller, C. (1988) Centralisation of treatments and survival rates for cancer. *Archives of Disease in Childhood*, **63**, 26.

Watson, M. (1983) Psychosocial interventions with cancer patients: a review. *Psychological Medicine*, **13**, 839–846.

Williams, E.M., Cruikshank, A. and Walker, W. (1972) Public opinion on cancer in S.E. Wales. Tenovus Cancer Information Centre, Cardiff.

2 | Staging investigations

As previously mentioned, the patient will undergo many investigations and staging procedures. The aim is to confirm the diagnosis and evaluate the spread of the disease. Accurate planning of the numerous procedures can prevent unnecessary trauma. The need for psychological preparation prior to investigations and treatments has been recognized in order to ensure that the child survives emotionally/psychologically as well as physically (Fotchman and Foley, 1982). Information booklets which illustrate procedures, clarify or back up verbal information may be of use to some children and families, but will be dependent upon the child's level of development and individual family members' needs.

Most investigations require the patient's co-operation, either to endure procedures that may require them to be in an uncomfortable position, separated from their carer or cope with an invasive assault on their body. It is important therefore to try and limit investigative programmes to those that are acceptable or tolerated by the patient and family.

Distress and anxieties experienced by children undergoing investigation and treatment for their cancer have been highlighted (Kratz, Kellerman and Siegal, 1980; Jay et al., 1983). They demonstrated that the age of the child can be a predictor to the level and intensity of distress and that younger children will show their distress more intensely. Preschool and school age children are usually open about their fears but adolescents' fear may be displayed by nausea, muscle tension and sweating. Girls display their fears more than boys, and although boys appeared to recover more quickly after procedures they were also more likely to try a stalling technique. The presence, support and reassurance of parents and physical contact with them during the procedure, e.g. hand holding, was reported by children with cancer as a coping strategy that helped make the procedure easier for them (Hamners and Miles, 1988).

The ability to cope with these invasive investigative procedures is dependent upon the development of effective coping strategies. Each child should be treated as an individual and with the parents be involved in the decision making and preparation for each of the procedures. There should not be preconceived expectations of children because of their age, disease or extent of their illness.

2.1 GENERAL ANAESTHESIA

Facilities for general anaesthesia are available in most paediatric oncology departments. They facilitate multiple invasive procedures, such as bone marrow aspirations, lumbar punctures, inspection and cleansing of wounds, change of dressings, insertion of cannulae, removal of sutures and insertion of catheters – urinary or nasogastric. Co-operation and communication between the ward and anaesthetic department personnel ensure appropriate equipment and adequate time are available.

'Loss of control' has been identified as one of five categories of adverse reactions to hospitalization (Muller, Harris and Wattley, 1986). Therefore the opportunity to choose the method of anaesthetic induction and the mode of transport to the department may help the patient cope with the procedures. The presence of the carer until the patient is anaesthetized has been demonstrated to be beneficial to both child and carer and admission to the anaesthetic room during induction is now a widely accepted practice.

2.2 LOCAL ANAESTHESIA

This may be in the form of injection or topical administration. Emla cream contains lignocaine and prilocaine and it is applied to the skin and left under a tagaderm dressing for a minimum of one hour. It is useful for the siting of needles, butterflies and cannulae and can also be used for facilitating the administration of intramuscular or subcutaneous injections. It is of particular use for a child whose medical condition contraindicates a general anaesthetic but who is unable to tolerate a local anaesthetic or other injection. Older children may find Entonox useful, both from its analgesic effect and diversional qualities.

2.3 SEDATION

Sedation may be required by children who are either anxious about forthcoming procedures or who are unable to comply with the requirements for the procedure, e.g. the required position for lumbar puncture or length of procedure, e.g. CT or MRI scanning.

Single agent sedatives are often not effective for the variety of procedures being performed. Often a combination of sedatives and analgesics is found to be very effective but may have the side effect of taking several hours for the child to awaken fully. When using this type of sedation cocktail it is advisable to timetable procedures/investigations for late afternoon, thus preventing the child sleeping for most of the day.

Medical procedures increase anxiety levels especially in young children. No one particular method of preparation is always suitable or effective (Kratz, Kellerman and Siegel, 1980). A flexible approach that allows and encourages children and their families to be treated as individuals will help to gain the child and family's trust and co-operation.

2.4 PREPARATION FOR SPECIFIC INVESTIGATIONS

Radiological Investigation. Plain X-rays still have an important role to play in diagnostic and staging investigations. They do not require any physical preparation and the psychological preparation will depend on the age of the child and any previous experience he may have had. Allowing the child time to be accustomed to the machinery, room and personnel will all help.

Computerized Axial Tomography Scanning (CAT or CT). Although not painful CT scans require a child to remain still for a period of time (this is dependent on the area or amount being scanned). Contrast medium to specify vessels or organs and to enhance normal tissue such as bowel may be given orally or intravenously. Oral contrast requires the patient to fast for two hours prior to the scan. The administration of the contrast requires patience and encouragement from parents and staff as it is not always possible to disguise the taste. The total volume of contrast may cause difficulties and if sedation is required to facilitate the scan, a nasogastric tube can be passed for its administration. CT scans of the chest require control of breathing, therefore if the patient is too young or unable to comply with controlled breathing intubation general anaesthesia is indicated. Where appropriate, other invasive, painful or threatening procedures may be planned and carried out under this anaesthetic.

MRI Scans. Although not painful MRI scans require the patient to lie still in a very restricting piece of equipment. Many patients, even adults, complain of feeling claustrophobic. Children may require sedation to facilitate this scan. Observing other children undergoing a scan or re-hearsing the procedure may be of use to some patients.

Nuclear Medicine Scans, e.g. ^{90}Tc bone scan, gallium scan. Venous access is required for the administration of the isotope. The scan itself is neither painful or threatening but does require the patient to lie still. A sedative cocktail will facilitate both the intravenous administration of the isotope and the scan itself.

Metaiodobenzylguanidine (mIBG). ^{123}I mIBG is administered intra-venously 24 hours prior to the scan. Uptake of the radioactive iodine by the thyroid is prevented by oral administration of iodine either as Lugol's iodine or potassium iodide tablets 48 hours prior to the administration of the MIBG. Radiation protection when handling excreta from the patient undergoing an MIBG scan is not required as the level of radioactivity is minimal. Preparation is as for any other isotope scan.

Diagnostic Ultrasound. Generally ultrasound scans are non-invasive and non-threatening, however, if there is swelling or distension at the tumour site a feeling of pressure or discomfort may be experienced – analgesia with or without sedation may therefore be required.

2.5 HAEMATOLOGICAL INVESTIGATIONS

Regular blood counts are one of the most common tests that children with cancer undergo. Although some children can cope or learn to cope with venepuncture or finger prick not all will. The first occasion on which each procedure is carried out constitutes a particularly important learning experience for that child. It is important therefore that the first approach is planned, taking the child's age, level of development and previous experience into consideration. The choice between finger prick (often very uncomfortable) and venepuncture should be left up to the child. The former is often used to facilitate rapid turnover rather than patient choice.

As previously mentioned, sedation is extremely useful and when used in this setting allows time for the most suitable vein to be identified without increasing the anxiety level in the child. Whenever possible choosing the non-dominant limb makes it easier for the child to continue to participate in daily activities.

Central venous catheters should be considered for children who are facing intensive chemotherapy regimens. Hickman lines, Broviac lines and Portacaths have individual advantages and disadvantages. The complexity of the chemotherapy protocol may be the deciding factor. Some of the intensive regimens now necessitate triple lumen venous access, while others are managed adequately with Portacaths or single lumen central lines.

The insertion of the central venous device requires careful preparation and planning. It may be possible to insert such a device during, or as part of, the investigative procedures. This will facilitate many of the remaining investigations and diagnostic tests and may prevent delay in the commencement of treatment once the diagnosis is confirmed.

The child and family will require advice as to the reason for the insertion of such a device, the advantages, disadvantages and alternatives. It may be appropriate for the child and family to state their preference for the device but as previously mentioned this may be determined by the patient's diagnosis and probable treatment protocol.

The play therapist again has a vital role to play in preparing the child or adolescent for the procedure. Using dolls that are anatomically correct may help the parents and child understand the placement of such a device. Observing and talking to other children and their parents may be helpful.

Injections have been identified as being one of the worst pains in cancer and therefore children are usually very happy to discuss and demonstrate the advantages and give advice as to the care of it. Older children and adolescents prefer Portacaths because the degree of altered body image is less. With any catheter a discussion with the surgeon regarding the exit site of the lines may be of great value to the patient. The ultimate scar should be as cosmetically acceptable as possible. Following the insertion of the central venous device the family and patient require information and demonstration of how to care for it at home. The timing of this must be carefully planned to avoid presenting the parents with too much information too soon but allowing them sufficient time to practise and gain confidence.

The information should be supported by written material (Wong and Whaley, 1990). It has been suggested that the initial demonstration to the parents of younger children is best carried out away from the child, to allow the parents to focus on the basic principles (Marcoux, Fisher and Wong, 1990). To avoid one parent carrying all the responsibility it is advisable to teach at least two family members. Practising on a model helps parents to overcome their anxieties and build up confidence without having the pressure of practising on their child. Supportive supervision should be offered until the parents are confident.

The patient's age and level of development will determine his/her participation in caring for the central venous device. As with the parents, they require detailed explanations of the care required. Information should include dressing changes, observations for infection or movement of the catheter, cleansing of the site, frequency of flushes and cap/bung changes. Advice should also be given regarding unusual occurrences, such as inability to flush the line, displacement of the line, emergence of the cuff, air in the line, displacement of the cap/bung or appearance of a split or leak in the catheter.

If the child is returning to school the teachers and school nurses should receive instruction and advice to prepare them to support the child (Dufour, 1990). Contact telephone numbers for the parents and school are invaluable.

It is useful to discuss with parents the practicalities of the most appropriate time and place to carry out this procedure at home. They may also require advice on storage and disposal of equipment.

2.6 RELAXATION TECHNIQUES

Stress during investigative and treatment procedures is the result of a child's perception of the situation as threatening (Hockenberry, 1988).

The child feels controlled by the situation rather than being in control. Relaxation can help to give an alternative perception to painful or invasive procedures. It can also help to control fear and discomfort, decrease side effects from the treatment and give the patient the opportunity to actively participate in his own care.

Parents and children can be taught relaxation techniques. The nurse's role is to support and educate the child and family as they develop effective coping mechanisms. Many parents find participating in their child's relaxation or diversional techniques beneficial and enable them to cope with the experience of watching their child undergo a traumatic procedure (Hockenberry, 1988).

Distraction is a method used regularly by parents and health care professionals. Glove puppets, favourite toys, books, story tapes, waving coloured objects are used to divert the patient's attention from the procedure. Older children find concentrating on their breathing – deep breaths in through their nose and exhaling through their mouth or holding their breath a helpful form of distraction and a way to participate by determining when to breathe. Imagery encourages the child to focus on pictures formed in their mind. It may be pleasant events that have happened in the past or visits to special places. Time must be spent prior to this method to discover the child's interests and likes. Muscle relaxation is a form of relaxation to decrease mental and physical tension. The patients are taught to first tense and then relax specific muscles. Control of breathing is also involved and it is used most effectively by adolescents. Hypnosis should be used by experienced professionals only; this is a combination of the previously mentioned methods to induce a more relaxed state. Again parent participation can be beneficial to both the child and family. Children have a natural ability to fantasize and imagine and appear to be more trusting than adults.

In conclusion, it is clear that the first few days whilst awaiting results are particularly stressful (Wilson Barnett and Carrigy, 1978). The need for information, advice and explanation is particularly acute.

The psychological care and support received by the child and family during the diagnostic phase has a major impact and will affect their ability to survive emotionally once the diagnosis is confirmed and treatment commences (Kratz, Kellerman and Sicgcl, 1980).

REFERENCES

Dufour, D.T. (1990) Information for teachers of children with central venous catheters. *Journal of Paediatric and Oncologic Nursing*, **7**(1), 37–38.
Fotchman, D. and Foley, G. (1982) *Nursing Care of the Child with Cancer*. Little Brown, Boston.
Hamners, B. and Miles, M.S. (1988) Coping strategies in children with cancer

undergoing bone marrow aspirations. *Journal of American Pediatric Oncology Nursing*, **5**(3), 11–14.

Hockenberry, M.J. (1988) Relaxation techniques in children with cancer. The nurse's role. *Journal of American Pediatric Oncology Nursing*, **5**(1,2), 7–11.

Jay, S.M., Ozolins, M., Elliotts, C.M. and Caldwell, S. (1983) Assessment of children's distress during painful medical procedures. *Health Psychology*, **2**, 133–147.

Kratz, E.R., Kellerman, J. and Siegel, S.E. (1980) Behavioral distress in children with cancer undergoing medical procedures – developmental considerations. *Journal of Consulting and Clinical Psychology*, **48**(3), 356–365.

Marcoux, C., Fisher, S. and Wong, D. (1990) Central venous devices in children. *Paediatric Nursing*, **16**(2), 123–132.

Muller, D.J., Harris, P.J. and Wattley, L. (1986) *The Effect of Hospitalisation on Children Nursing Children, Psychology Research & Practice*, Chapman and Hall, London.

Wilson Barnett, J. and Carrigy, A. (1978) Factors influencing patients' emotional reactions to hospitalisation. *Journal of Advanced Nursing*, **3**, 221–229.

Wong, D. and Whaley, L.F. (1990) *Clinical Manual of Paediatric Nursing*, 3rd edn, C.V. Mosby, St Louis.

Making a clinical and pathological diagnosis

3

3.1 MAKING A CLINICAL DIAGNOSIS

Initial clinical examination, often in the out-patients department, will give a strong clue as to the nature of the disease and a number of simple non-invasive diagnostic procedures will further narrow down the differential diagnosis. Specific diagnostic procedures are described in detail under the individual cancer types. In Table 3.1 the differential diagnoses of a thoracic mass evaluated by chest X-ray are shown.

Abdominal ultrasound has become an invaluable diagnostic tool in the assessment of children's cancer. This technique often requires no sedation, even in a small child, and will provide information regarding the organ of origin of the tumour, associated nodal involvement and any vascular invasion (Figure 3.1). The evolution of high resolution colour Doppler ultrasound machines has made this the investigation of choice in detecting and assessing intravascular invasion, for example, in Wilms' tumour or hepatoblastoma. Table 3.2 lists the likely diagnoses following initial abdominal localization.

Thoracic ultrasound may be of value in distinguishing a pleural effusion from a solid mass or consolidation, which may be difficult on plain X-ray or even CT scan. In the investigation of jaundice, ultrasound will detect metastatic disease in the liver, large vessel thrombosis or intrahepatic candidiasis. It may also reveal fungal lesions in the spleen. Ultrasound of the testes can be of value in confirming clinically suspicious infiltration in leukaemia or lymphoma. The nature of other soft tissue masses may be clarified by ultrasound, such as benign lesions like cystic hygroma or varicocele.

Other radiological imaging

Plain X-ray of the abdomen may demonstrate intratumoural calcification. This is typical of neuroblastoma but also occurs in malignant or benign germ cell tumours. It is very rarely seen in other abdominal tumours.

Table 3.1 Differential diagnoses of thoracic mass evaluated by P.A. and lateral chest X-ray

	Anterior mediastinal	Posterior mediastinal
Malignant	Non-Hodgkin's lymphoma Hodgkin's lymphoma Malignant germ cell tumour Rhabdomyosarcoma, Ewing's sarcoma Thymoma	Neuroblastoma Ganglioneuroblastoma Sarcoma Phaeochromocytoma
Benign	Teratoma Cystic hygroma Haemangioma Thymic cyst	Ganglioneuroma Schwann cell tumour Neurofibroma Bronchogenic cyst

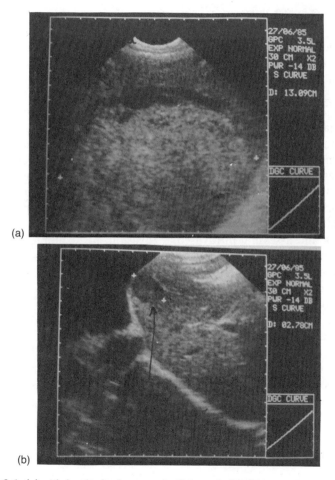

(a)

(b)

Figure 3.1 (a) Abdominal ultrasound of large adrenal neuroblastoma showing lifting of vena cava anteriorly. (b) Ultrasound of liver in child with Wilms' tumour showing hepatic metastasis.

Table 3.2 Differential diagnoses of abdominal mass after initial localization using ultrasound examination

Renal	Suprarenal	Hepatic	Intestinal	Pelvic

Wilms' tumour
Renal carcinoma
	Neuroblastoma
	Polar Wilms'
		Hepatoblastoma
		Hepatic carcinoma
			Lymphoma
			Rhabdomyosarcoma
				Germ cell tumour
				Rhabdomyosarcoma
				of: uterus
				    vagina
				    prostate

Mesoblastic nephroma	Hepatic tumour	Rhabdomyosarcoma	Soft tissue sarcoma Ewing's sarcoma	
Intrarenal neuroblastoma	Adrenal carcinoma	Angiosarcoma	Nodal metastases	Ewing's sarcoma – soft tissue or bone Osteosarcoma
Teratoma Lymphoma/leukaemia	Phaeochromocytoma	Cholangiosarcoma Teratoma Metastatic tumour		Neuroblastoma Metastatic nodes Ovarian cyst
Abscess Granuloma	Focal nodular hyperplasia Hydatid cyst	Haemangioma Appendix abscess Lipoma Pancreatic pseudocyst	Mesenteric cyst Haematocolpos Pelvic abscess	

Calcification will, however, also be apparent on CT scan and abdominal plain X-rays are therefore rarely used. Plain X-ray of bone is of great value in the differential diagnosis of primary bone tumours. The nature of bone destruction, whether cystic or diffuse, the pattern of extension through periosteum and any soft tissue infiltration are all useful clues. A large calcified soft tissue mass is much more likely in osteosarcoma (Figure 3.2) than in Ewing's sarcoma where the tumour may be confined to the bone often with only a lytic lesion and some periosteal elevation.

Skeletal surveys are now rarely performed and have been largely superseded by [99]technetium bone scan. The one exception is Langerhans' cell histiocytosis where in the routine initial staging the skeletal survey is retained as it has been shown to be more sensitive than isotope bone scan. Plain X-ray of skull is of importance with soft tissue sarcomas or lymphomas involving this area as bony erosion may upstage the patient and necessitate more intensive chemotherapy or the addition of radiotherapy.

Intravenous pyelograms are still recommended in some centres for the assessment of Wilms' tumour. Their main value is to demonstrate a normal functioning contralateral kidney which is important prior to nephrectomy. However, good quality ultrasound will provide this information and also give more useful imaging of the tumour itself compared to the pyelogram.

Lymphography has now little role in paediatric cancer. In the past it was used routinely for children with paratesticular rhabdomyosarcoma and those with Hodgkin's lymphoma. It has been superseded by high resolution CT scanning of abdominal nodes. Occasionally in the older child where lymphography is technically feasible, it may be used where the CT scan result is equivocal.

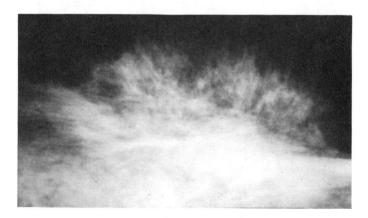

Figure 3.2 Typical sunburst appearance of plain X-ray associated with soft tissue calcification in osteogenic sarcoma.

CT scanning

This imaging modality more than any other plays a definitive role in the documentation of the extent of the primary tumour and in the accurate assessment of tumour response. Most chemotherapy studies require regular reassessment of tumour bulk and accurate two- or three-dimensional measurement to determine both the effectiveness of therapy and the possible prognostic importance of initial speed of response (Figure 3.3).

CT scan will give information regarding the local extent of tumour in virtually any part of the body. As mentioned above it is now used routinely to detect abdominal nodal involvement. It is also used to detect small bulk lung metastases not evident on chest X-ray. CT scan of chest is mandatory in the initial staging of osteosarcoma, Ewing's sarcoma, hepatic tumour, germ cell tumour and Wilms' tumour if the chest X-ray is negative. Imaging of bony tumours will provide additional information to the plain X-ray and delineates more clearly the extent of any adjacent soft tissue mass (Figure 3.4).

With most children under the age of three years sedation or general anaesthesia is required for adequate CT scanning. When imaging the lungs a general anaesthesia may be preferable to enable control of inspiration.

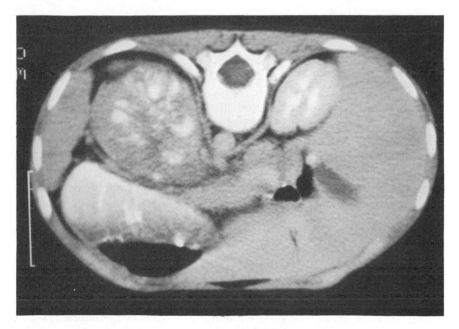

Figure 3.3 Abdominal CT scan showing heavily calcified right adrenal neuroblastoma.

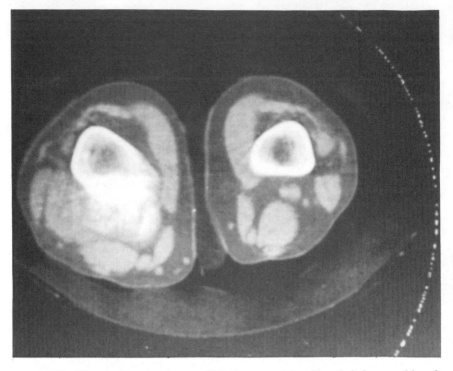

Figure 3.4 CT scan showing large calcified mass arising from left femur with soft tissue calcification due to osteogenic sarcoma.

Magnetic resonance imaging

This modality is increasingly used in the evaluation of tumour extent. Although it provides anatomically impressive pictures only in a minority of situations it is superior to CT scanning in terms of the information provided. An example of this is the delineation of brain tumours in the posterior fossa or base of skull region where bony artefact may compromise the quality of CT scans. MRI has also largely replaced the need for myelography or CT myelograms in the assessment of either primary spinal tumours or intraspinal extension from neuroblastoma or primitive neuro-ectodermal tumours (Figure 3.5). In the staging of brain tumours which seed into the spinal fluid, such as medulloblastoma, there is as yet insufficient data supporting the use of MRI alone to replace routine CSF cytological examination and myelography.

The character of the MRI signal may be of value in determining the nature of some soft tissue tumours and also may detect minimal residual disease more accurately than CT scan. The latter is the subject of a number of prospective studies in tumours such as Ewing's sarcoma,

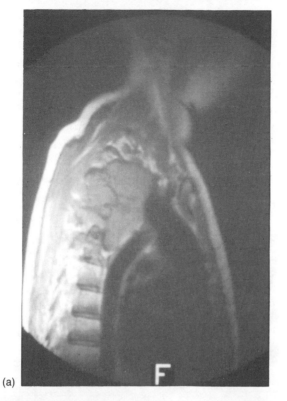

(a)

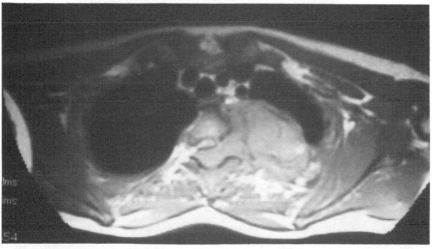

(b)

Figure 3.5 (a) Sagittal and (b) transverse MRI scans showing a posterior mediastinal mass infiltrating into spinal canal. This child with neuroblastoma presented
with clinical signs of cord compression.

rhabdomyosarcoma and neuroblastoma (Figure 3.6). MRI will elegantly demonstrate bone marrow involvement in neuroblastoma but less accurately than ^{123}I metaiodobenzylguanidine (mIBG) scanning. It will also demonstrate marrow involvement in lymphoproliferative disease and other solid tumour metastases (Figure 3.7). One limitation in the younger child is the time taken for the scan and therefore the need for heavy sedation during the scanning period. General anaesthesia is technically a problem due to the need to exclude all metals from the machine field.

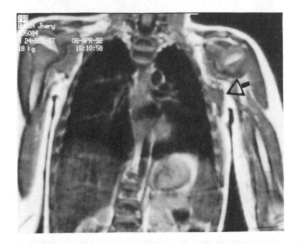

Figure 3.6 MRI scan of recurrent nodal disease in child with rhabdomyosarcoma of the left forearm.

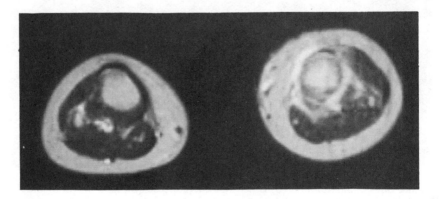

Figure 3.7 MRI scan of tibia showing abnormal high signal associated with marrow involvement. There is also soft tissue infiltration adjacent to bone.

Isotope scanning

As mentioned above [99]technetium scanning has largely replaced X-rays in the staging of tumours which metastasize to bone. These include neuroblastoma, rhabdomyosarcoma, Ewing's sarcoma and osteogenic sarcoma. It is worth noting that technetium is also taken up by the primary tumour in neuroblastoma (Figure 3.8).

[67]Gallium imaging of lymph nodes is currently under evaluation in Hodgkin's disease and non-Hodgkin's lymphoma. Isotope is taken up by lymph nodes which are either infected or involved with tumour whereas residual post-treatment fibrotic nodes are negative. Unfortunately gallium is also taken up by the thymus and thymic hyperplasia may occur at unpredictable stages during chemotherapy or following cessation of chemotherapy. It is important therefore to correlate gallium uptake with imaging of the thymus either using CT scan or MRI (Figure 3.9).

Tumour specific imaging

Metaiodobenzylguanidine (mIBG) structurally resembles the adrenergic neurone blocker guanethidine and the neurotransmitter noradrenaline and is taken up by adrenal medulla and tumours of sympathetic nervous system origin. It is therefore a useful imaging agent in phaeochromo-

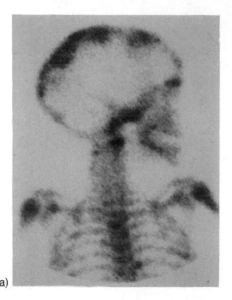
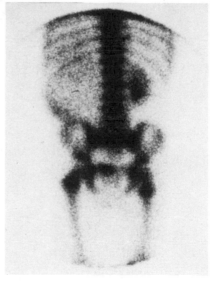

(a) (b)

Figure 3.8 (a) Technetium bone scan showing multiple bony abnormalities particularly in the vault of the skull. (b) Technetium scan showing uptake in the left-sided suprarenal primary.

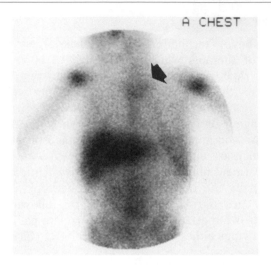

Figure 3.9 Increased gallium uptake in mediastinal mass of Hodgkin's disease.

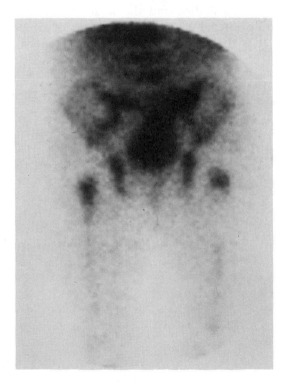

Figure 3.10 Multiple abnormal foci of uptake in femora, pelvis and spine in metastatic neuroblastoma.

cytoma (which is extremely rare in children) and neuroblastoma. A number of iodine isotopes have been used to label mIBG such as ^{125}I, ^{131}I and ^{123}I. ^{123}I is the isotope of choice for routine tumour imaging and has been shown to clearly demonstrate both primary tumour and distant metastases in the majority of patients with stage 4 disease (Figure 3.10). There is general consensus now that this is the most sensitive way of detecting minimal distant disease in bone marrow. There is, however, some controversy regarding its ability to distinguish patchy bone from patchy bone marrow disease.

3.2 MAKING A PATHOLOGICAL DIAGNOSIS

It is self-evident that accurate pathological diagnosis is of paramount importance in the management of children's cancer. Treatment intensity and nature varies widely in both solid tumours and haemopoietic malignancies, depending on the nature of the tumour. Although a diagnosis may be made within 24 hours in the case of leukacmia, with solid tumours this may take several days. This is a difficult waiting period for the patient and family but it must be emphasized to them the importance of being absolutely confident of the precise nature of the cancer.

Leukaemias and lymphomas

An initial bone marrow sample is taken by aspiration either under local anaesthetic or with short acting intravenous or inhalation anaesthesia. Under the same procedure a cerebrospinal fluid sample is taken. Because of potentially patchy involvement trephine biopsy is usually taken with lymphomas and may be necessary in some cases of leukaemia where aspiration is difficult. A so-called 'dry tap' is not uncommon where the marrow is packed with tumour cells. A slide preparation taken from a trephine biopsy (roll prep.) may be of value and will provide cells for immunophenotyping, often more limited using fixed trephine tissue.

The usual site of marrow aspiration in a child is the posterior iliac crest although the anterior crest may also be used. It is rarely necessary to use the sternal or tibial sites, although occasionally the tibia may be appropriate in a small infant.

Morphological and immunophenotypic studies done on the marrow from non-Hodgkin's lymphoma are essentially the same as those used for the leukaemias. Morphological classification of leukaemias is based on the Franco–American–British (FAB) classification, Table 3.3. Details of leukaemia immunophenotyping are given in Chapter 9.

Table 3.3 FAB classification of lymphoblastic leukaemia

Cytologic features	L1	L2	L3
Cell size	Small	Large	Large and homogeneous
Nuclear chromatin	Homogeneous	Variable, heterogeneous	Finely stippled and homogeneous
Nuclear shape	Regular, occasional clefting	Irregular, clefting and indentation common	Regular – oval to round
Nucleoli	Not visible or small and inconspicuous	One or more present, often large	Prominent, one or more
Amount of cytoplasm	Scanty	Variable	Moderately abundant
Basophilia of cytoplasm	Slight or moderate	Variable	Deep
Cytoplasmic vacuolation	Variable	Variable	Prominent

Solid tumours

The diagnosis usually rests on tissue biopsy from the primary tumour site. In the case of lymphomas, however, examination of ascitic fluid or pleural effusion may produce sufficient cells for detailed morphological and immunophenotyping and preclude the need for further tissue sampling. This is rarely the case in other solid tumours.

In tumours with markers such as neuroblastoma (urinary catecholamines) or hepatoblastoma and germ cell tumours (alpha-fetoprotein, beta-HCG) the diagnosis may be almost certain on the basis of marker positivity and primary tumour imaging. However, in general, tissue biopsy is mandatory. With increasing evidence that biological characteristics are of prognostic importance it is essential that sufficient tissue is obtained for such analysis. Fine needle biopsies are usually inadequate

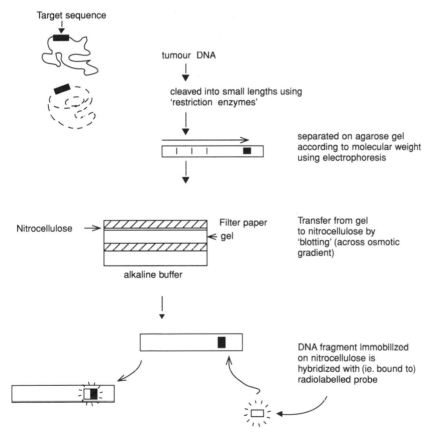

Figure 3.11 Southern blot preparation of DNA.

but multiple Trucut biopsy where several cores of tissue are obtained is an alternative to open biopsy.

Some of the special stains used in differentiating small round cell tumours are shown below:

Leucocyte common antigen	Haemopoietic e.g. NHL
Desmin Myoglobin	Rhabdomyosarcoma
Neurone specific enolase	Neuroblastoma, Ewing's, PNET
PGP 1.5	Neuroblastoma, Ewing's, PNET

These include a number of monoclonal antibody preparations. These are antibodies which are raised specifically against a structure present on the surface or in the cytoplasm of the tumour cells. Although these are often

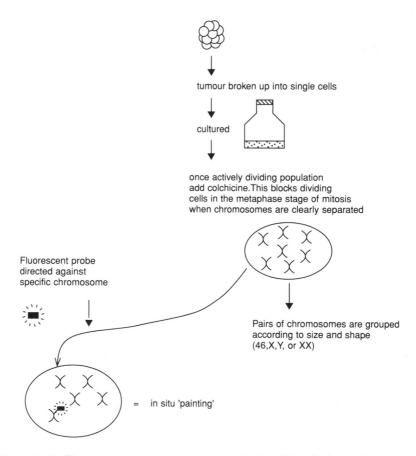

tumour broken up into single cells

cultured

once actively dividing population
add colchicine.This blocks dividing
cells in the metaphase stage of mitosis
when chromosomes are clearly separated

Fluorescent probe
directed against
specific chromosome

Pairs of chromosomes are grouped
according to size and shape
(46,X,Y, or XX)

= in situ 'painting'

Figure 3.12 Chromosome preparation and *in situ* labelling ('painting').

not absolutely tumour specific if a panel of antibodies are positive this will provide strong evidence of one type of tumour.

Increasingly, molecular biological techniques are used in the initial diagnosis of tumours. DNA isolated from tumour cells can be labelled with probes (specific base sequences complementary to the base sequence in question). The DNA is denatured and separated on the basis of molecular weight by electrophoresis on a gel and then the probe is added. The probe, if it is bound to the DNA, can be picked up either with special stains or radio-active labelling (southern blot) (Figure 3.11). Similar techniques can be used for staining RNA (northern blot) or whole protein (western blot).

Cytogenetics now plays an essential role in the initial evaluation of childhood leukaemia both in terms of classification of disease and prognosis. Although it is technically more difficult to isolate tumour karyotype from solid tissue, this is increasingly done and has achieved increasing importance. Figure 3.12 illustrates the isolation of a chromosome preparation.

Recently so-called 'chromosome painting' has been developed. In this technique fluorescent probes are constructed which because they have a complementary base sequence to the part of the chromosome of interest will bind with the relevant site. This may be of use in demonstrating translocations or deletions (Figure 3.12).

4 Epidemiology and aetiology of childhood cancer

Malignant disease is rare in childhood with an annual incidence of approximately 1 in 10 000 children under 15 years of age. A general practitioner would therefore see only 1–2 cases in a career and the general paediatrician a handful of cases every decade. None the less, it is the second commonest cause of non-accidental death in children.

The United Kingdom National Registry of Childhood Tumours based in Oxford receives notifications of the diagnoses of all children with cancer under the age of 15 years. This provides an invaluable database gathered over the last 30 years and is one of the few national unselected registers of this type. In Table 4.1 the annual incidences of haematological and solid tumours are listed and the sex ratio shown. The commonest group of diagnoses are the leukaemias, the majority of which are acute lymphoblastic leukaemia. Second largest group are the brain tumours, followed by soft tissue sarcomas and lymphomas.

Paediatric tumours can be divided into three broad groups:

1. Embryonal neoplasms. These are due to faulty development of embryonal cells, leading to a persistence and proliferation of cells closely resembling the fetal tissue.
2. Juvenile neoplasms. These arise due to malignant transformation in mature tissue cells but are prevalent in, or even unique to, the younger age group.
3. Adult-type tumours. These are tumours which are rarely seen in children and are histologically identical to adult counterparts.

These groups include the following:

Embryonal Tumours   *Adult-type*
Germ cell tumours
Nephroblastoma   Hepatocellular carcinoma
Neuroblastoma   Renal cell carcinoma
Medulloblastoma   Synovial cell carcinoma

Table 4.1 Annual incidence of childhood cancers in UK (National Registry data)

Diagnostic group	Annual rates per million	Sex ratio (M/F)
Total	106.7	1.3
I Leukaemias		
Acute lymphoblastic	29.7	1.4
Acute non-lymphoblastic	6.0	1.2
Chronic myeloid	0.8	1.4
II Lymphomas		
Hodgkin's disease	4.1	2.5
Non-Hodgkin	6.1	2.4
III Brain and spinal		
Ependymoma	3.1	1.3
Astrocytoma	8.9	1.1
Medulloblastoma	5.0	1.7
IV Sympathetic nervous system		
Neuroblastoma	7.0	1.4
V Retinoblastoma	3.5	1.0
VI Kidney		
Wilms' tumour	7.2	1.0
Renal carcinoma	0.1	1.7
VII Liver		
Hepatoblastoma	0.8	0.8
Hepatic carcinoma	0.2	1.4
VIII Bone		
Osteosarcoma	2.4	1.1
Ewing's sarcoma	1.7	1.2
IX Soft tissue sarcomas		
Rhabdomyosarcoma	4.2	1.6
Fibrosarcoma	0.8	1.0
X Gonadal and germ cell		
Non-gonadal germ cell	0.9	0.7
Gonadal germ cell	1.5	1.0
XI Epithelial		
Adrenocortical carcinoma	0.3	0.4
Thyroid carcinoma	0.3	0.4
Nasopharyngeal carcinoma	0.3	1.4

Rhabdomyosarcoma
Hepatoblastoma
Retinoblastoma
Primitive neuroectodermal tumour

Juvenile Neoplasms
Cerebral astrocytoma and ependymoma
Ewing's sarcoma

Schwannoma
Carcinoma, e.g. nasopharyngeal

Osteosarcoma
Non-Hodgkin's lymphoma
Hodgkin's lymphoma

Early age peaks in incidence are found in acute lymphoblastic leukaemia (ALL) and also embryonal tumours. In neuroblastoma, retinoblastoma and hepatoblastoma the highest incidence is in the first year of life. Other tumours, such as Hodgkin's disease, osteosarcoma and Ewing's sarcoma, show a peak in early adolescence which continues into early adulthood. As can be seen from Table 4.1 male sex predominates in the lymphomas, both Hodgkin's and non-Hodgkin's. With gonadal germ cell tumours there is an excess of girls limited only to the older age group.

Data comparing relative incidences of childhood cancer in different countries and between different races are difficult to interpret because of limitations regarding registration of diagnosis. Up until recently Wilms' tumour was thought to have a standard incidence worldwide and was therefore used as a yardstick for the quality of tumour registration. However, recently the incidence in Japan has been shown to be significantly lower than elsewhere. Within western countries differences between racial groups exist and are largely unexplained. For example a peak incidence in ALL between the age of 2–3 years is found in Caucasian Americans but not in Afro-Caribbean Americans.

A recent review of the incidence of childhood cancer amongst ethnic groups in the United Kingdom demonstrated a lower peak incidence early in life but no difference between Caucasian and Asian children. In contrast, there appeared to be a particularly high incidence of Hodgkin's disease amongst Asian children, particularly in the younger age group with predominance of the mixed cellularity subtypes. This is similar to the disease pattern in the Indian and African subcontinent and suggests that in this ethnic group aetiological factors persist despite the geographical variations. Wilms' tumour had a substantially higher relative frequency amongst older children in the West Indian population, whereas Asian children have a relatively low frequency. The absence of Ewing's sarcoma amongst West Indian children was also noted and was consistent with the low incidence of this tumour amongst black Americans (Stiller *et al.*, 1991).

4.1 ENVIRONMENTAL FACTORS

Because of the rarity of childhood cancer it is particularly difficult to draw firm conclusions regarding the impact of specific environmental factors on the incidence of any tumour. Being the commonest childhood cancer leukaemia has been the focus of most studies. It has been shown, however, that clusters of leukaemia may occur in areas purely by chance in the absence of any hypothesized risk factor.

Radiation exposure to the fetus *in utero* was shown over 30 years ago to increase the risk of acute leukaemia. Comparatively low doses of radiation given in the 1950s to treat scalp ringworm were shown to significantly increase the risk of a variety of neural tumours, despite the dose being only 1–2 Gy (Ron *et al.*, 1988). The impact of nuclear power generating plants on the incidence of leukaemia has been an area of hot debate over the last decade; one study has shown a significant increase in the incidence of leukaemia in a birth cohort of children born to mothers resident in Seascale, England, where the overall incidence of leukaemia aged under 10 years was several times the national average. A further study suggested that the causal factor was exposure of fathers to low dose ionizing radiation when they were employed at a nuclear plant. This contrasts with the absence of cancer risk in the offspring of those who were exposed to atomic bomb radiation. The precise mechanisms involved, with regard to radiation dose–time relationships are unclear (Gardner *et al.*, 1987, 1990; Alexander *et al.*, 1990). Exposure to ionizing radiation from the atomic bombs in Japan was followed by an increase in leukaemias which peaked around five years after exposure. It is likely a similar phenomenon is now being observed in the Soviet republics following the Chernobyl accident.

The issue regarding clustering around nuclear power plants is complex and other hypotheses to explain a possible increase include the influx of population into a previously unpopulated area. This could have the effect of introducing viral pathogens to which the endogenous population had not been exposed, which caused the malignancy (Kinlen, 1990). The nature of such a viral infection is, however, unknown and unproven. The influence of background irradiation, particularly that of radon, and electromagnetic field have recently come under scrutiny (Cartwright, 1989; Henshaw, Eatough & Richardson, 1990).

It is hoped that the recently commenced United Kingdom national case control study of childhood cancers will throw light on some of these factors. In this study all children with haematological or solid malignancies will be investigated with regard to family history and environmental factors. These will be compared with age matched control children.

The only two drugs which have been shown to be associated with a significantly higher incidence of childhood cancer are diethylstilboestrol, which was linked with vaginal carcinoma and nitrosamines, which have been linked with brain tumours (Preston-Martin *et al.*, 1982). There are small case controlled reports suggesting correlations with a wide range of other agents, such as phenytoin, barbiturates and diuretics but these have not been substantiated (Stiller, 1991). Chloramphenicol, which is now rarely used in children, may increase the risk of acute leukaemia (Shu *et al.*, 1988). Similarly, a variety of chemicals, including pesticides, hair dye and marijuana have been implicated but remain unproven. Prolonged treatment with androgens in Fanconi's anaemia is linked with an increased incidence of hepatoblastoma.

Cytotoxic agents, in particular the alkylating agents, such as cyclophosphamide and CCNU are associated with an increased incidence of malignancy, especially myeloid leukaemia. More recently the epipodophyllotoxin, teniposide, when given weekly has been implicated in the induction of myeloid leukaemia, particularly associated with abnormalities of chromosome 11q:23.

4.2 ROLE OF INFECTION

The role played by Epstein–Barr virus (EBV) in the evolution of a number of neoplasms has undergone considerable study. Nasopharyngeal carcinoma and Burkitt's lymphoma are the best known examples. The molecular basis of B cell non-Hodgkin's lymphoma (NHL), including Burkitt's lymphoma, is discussed later but it appears that EBV may play a role by immortalising (i.e. inducing the ability of the cell to self-replicate) cells which have undergone spontaneous cytogenetic mutations. The latter are the basis of growth disregulation. Following organ transplants such as liver, heart/lung and kidney, persisting EBV infections may be associated with lymphoma-like lymphoproliferative disorders or even high grade B cell NHL (Penn, 1990; Swinnen et al., 1990).

Although the majority of children with hepatocellular carcinoma do not have any previous history of hepatitis B this link may exist.

An indirect association between infection and leukaemia has been proposed by Greaves and Chan (1986) and Greaves (1988). It is postulated that the rapid proliferation of the B cell population in utero leads to a spontaneous mutation (as opposed to a mutation transmitted in the germ line or induced by carcinogenic agents). The second event leading to overt leukaemia occurs at a time of subsequent maximum proliferative stress on lymphocyte precursor population, i.e. in early infancy.

There has been much speculation about the role of a viral pathogen in Hodgkin's disease. It is of interest that in underdeveloped countries where rates of infection in infancy are high the age of onset of Hodgkin's disease is much lower than in western countries and the tumour tends to be of mixed cellularity, rather than nodular sclerosing. It has been suggested that the later onset of Hodgkin's in western countries is due to a lack of early exposure to the pathogen. This failure to develop immunity results in the lymphoma following late exposure.

The influence of early breast feeding may be linked with patterns of virus infection. Prolonged breast feeding may reduce the relative risk for

ALL and for lymphomas. These data are, however, equivocal (Davis, Savitz and Graubard, 1988).

4.3 GENETIC FACTORS

Structural chromosome abnormalities are often found in tumour cells but this may reflect the instability of a rapidly dividing cell population rather than any primary defect involved in pathogenesis (Table 4.2).

In Table 4.3 a number of inherited diseases are shown which are associated with an increased incidence of malignancies. For the majority of these the mechanisms are not understood (Levine, King and Bloomfield, 1989; Ponder, 1991).

Retinoblastoma is the only childhood tumour where there is often a strong family history and the tumour can be traced back in about one-third cases. In Wilms' tumour there may be a family history in about 1% of cases. Aggregations of tumour within families have been reported in both neuroblastoma and hepatoblastoma but these are unusual. With other tumours the risk to a sibling is about double that of the normal population but this risk is still very low and rarely justifies any screening of siblings. In general parents are reassured that the risks are negligible. In neurofibromatosis (Von Recklinghausen's disease) there is an increased risk of

Table 4.2 Chromosomal abnormalities associated with specific malignancies

Chromosomal abnormalities	Malignancy
t(8;21), (15;17)	Acute myeloid leukaemia
t(8;22), (8;14), (2;8)	B cell leukaemia and lymphoma
t(4;11)	High count ALL, especially infants
t(1;19)	Pre-B ALL
t(11;14)	T cell ALL
t(9;22)	Chronic myeloblastic leukaemia
Monosomy 7	Myelodysplastic syndrome
Deletion 11p	Wilms' tumour
Deletion 13q	Retinoblastoma, osteosarcoma
t(11;22)	Ewing's sarcoma and primitive neuroectodermal tumour
t(2;13)	Alveolar rhabdomyosarcoma
Deletion 1p	Neuroblastoma
Deletion 6q 21	Large cell anaplastic lymphoma
Inversion 17q	Astrocytoma
Inversion 12p	Germ cell tumour
Deletion 22q	Meningioma
t(x;11)	Synovial sarcoma

Table 4.3 Inherited diseases which are associated with an increased incidence of malignancy

Primary disease	Inheritance	Predisposed tumour
Neurofibromatosis	AD	Sarcoma, neuroma, meningioma, glioma, phaeochromocytoma, leukaemia
Tuberous sclerosis	AD	Fibroma, cardiac rhabdomyosarcoma
Von Hippel–Lindau's syndrome	AD/AR	Retinal and cerebellar angioma, phaeochromocytoma, hypernephroma
Multiple endocrine neoplasia syndromes	AD	Pancreatic, adrenal, pituitary, parathyroid adenoma, schwannoma, medullary carcinoma of thyroid, phaeochromocytoma, neurofibroma
Naevoid basal cell carcinoma	AD	Basal cell carcinoma, medulloblastoma
Familial polyposis coli	AD	Colonic carcinoma
Peutz–Jegher	AD	Ovarian granulosa cell sarcoma
Haemochromatosis	AD/AR	Hepatocellular carcinoma
Multiple exostosis	AD	Osteosarcoma, chondrosarcoma
Fibro-osseous dysplasia	AD	Osteosarcoma, medullary fibrosarcoma
Kostmann's syndrome	AR	Monocytic leukaemia
Bruton's disease	XR	Leukaemia, lymphoma
Wiskott–Aldrich syndrome		
Ataxia telangiectasia	AR	Leukaemia, lymphoma, glioma
Bloom's syndrome	AR	Leukaemia, GIT
Fanconi's disease	AR	Acute myeloid leukaemia, hepatocarcinoma
Dyskeratosis congenita	XR	Squamous cell carcinoma
Beckwith's syndrome	AR	Adrenal carcinoma, Wilms' tumour
Tyrosinaemia, galactosaemia Wilson's syndrome, alpha-1 antitrypsin	AR	Hepatoma

AD = Autosomal dominant   GIT = gastrointestinal tract
AR = Autosomal recessive
XR = X-linked recessive

CNS tumours, particularly optic nerve glioma, fibrosarcoma and chronic myeloid leukaemia.

One familial cancer syndrome which has been of particular interest in recent years is the Li–Fraumeni syndrome, in which the occurrence of childhood rhabdomyosarcoma is associated with a high risk of breast cancer in the mother (Li & Fraumeni, 1969). In these families there is also an abnormally high incidence of other soft tissue sarcomas, adrenocortical carcinoma and CNS tumours. The risk of osteosarcoma, lung cancer and laryngeal carcinoma may also be increased. It has been suggested that up to 1% of all childhood cancers are part of the Li–Fraumeni syndrome.

Rarely the chromosome abnormalities are detectable in the normal cell population and this predisposes to cancer in a particular tissue. Retinoblastoma is the classic example; 30% of retinoblastomas have a family history and in about 5% peripheral lymphocyte chromosomes show a visible deletion of a variable portion of chromosome 13 always involving the q14 region. Large visible deletions tend to be associated with other phenotypic abnormalities, such as hypertelorism, micrognathia, a long philtrum, bulbous nose and mental retardation. Small deletions will be transmitted by an affected parent but can only be detected by using new molecular probes.

Chromosome 13 deletions are found in the tumour tissue in a high percentage of retinoblastoma patients who have normal somatic chromosomes and it has become clear that this is the site of the retinoblastoma gene. The 13q 14 deletion is found in tumour tissue from both familial and sporadic retinoblastoma.

Three major molecular mechanisms have been proposed for the development of childhood cancer. These are: loss of a tumour suppressor gene, leading to uncontrolled cell division; translocation of an oncogene to a site which influences its function, and thirdly mutation of a growth regulatory gene, such as p53 (Weinberg, 1989; Israel, 1992).

An oncogene or proto-oncogene is a gene normally found in human cells which is structurally similar to a viral gene that is capable of causing malignant transformation when inserted in experimental tissue. In man these genes may have a growth regulatory function which is upset by changes in the gene (Figure 4.1). Some of the specific oncogenes that may be abnormal in childhood tumours are shown in Table 4.4. The influence of the loss of a tumour suppressor gene is summarized in Figure 4.2 and this mechanism has been postulated for retinoblastoma (chromosome 13q 14) and Wilms' tumour (chromosome 11p 13). The Knudson 'Two hit' hypothesis suggests that two mutational events are necessary for tumour development. Each mutation results in the inactivation of identical genetic loci on each allele of chromosome 13 leading to a complete loss of normal genetic information from that gene. In familial retinoblastoma the first mutation, usually a deletion or point mutation, arises as a germ cell mutation in an otherwise normal individual. This mutation is then transmitted to an offspring who will therefore carry the mutation in all somatic cells. The second event is a mutation occurring specifically in a retinal cell

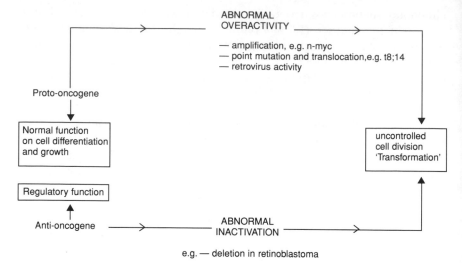

Figure 4.1 Gene regulation and oncogenesis.

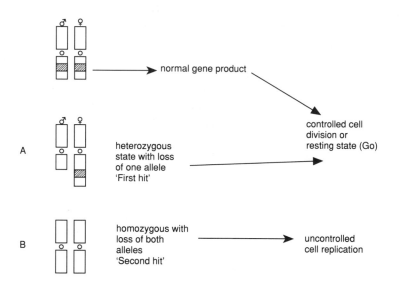

Figure 4.2 Loss of tumour suppressor gene ('Two hit' hypothesis).

Table 4.4 Oncogenes implicated in childhood tumours

Group	Location of gene product	Tumour
Protein kinases	Plasma membrane	
SRC		Sarcoma
abl		CML, ALL
erb b		Glioma
Growth factors		
Sis	Cytoplasm	Sarcoma
Ras family		
N-ras	Plasma membrane	Neuroblastoma
H/K ras		Neuroblastoma
		Rhabdomyosarcoma
Nuclear protein family		
N-myc	Nucleus	Neuroblastoma
C-myc		B NHL
		PNET

or cells which affects the other previously normal allele and this initiates tumour development.

In sporadic retinoblastoma both mutations occur as somatic events in retinal cells but again must affect both alleles at the appropriate locus on chromosome 13. Familial retinoblastoma occurs at a younger age and is often bilateral, due to the pre-existing predisposing mutation on one allele.

Other tumours in which the loss of a suppressor gene may be involved are listed below:

1p	Neuroblastoma
3p	Renal carcinoma, small cell lung carcinoma
5q	Colon carcinoma
11p	Wilms' tumour, bladder carcinoma
13q	Retinoblastoma
22q	Acoustic neuroma (NF2)

Chromosome translocation with juxtaposition of an oncogene has been described in B lymphoblastic lymphoma (Burkitt's and non-Burkitt's) involving the c-myc gene on chromosome 8 which is juxtaposed to the immunoglobulin heavy chain locus in chromosome 14 or the kappa and lambda light chain gene loci on chromosomes 2 and 22 respectively. This translocation appears to influence the function of c-myc oncogene, although the precise mechanism of this is unclear (Figure 4.3). In the case of chronic myeloid leukaemia and rare forms of acute lymphoblastic

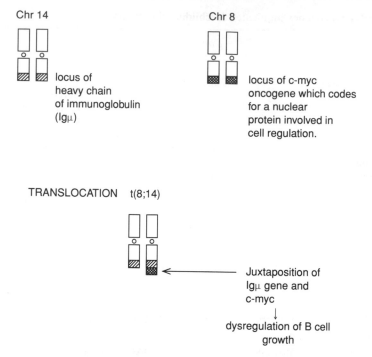

Figure 4.3 Translocation of oncogene resulting in functional alteration/activation.

leukaemia the c-abl oncogene on chromosome 9 is juxtaposed with the bcr gene on chromosome 22, resulting in the formation of the Philadelphia chromosome. The Ph chromosome found in ALL differs from chronic granulocytic leukaemia (CGL) only at a molecular level with regard to the precise nature of the translocation site.

The p53 gene has been described as 'the guardian of the genome' (Lane, 1992). It has been suggested that it plays a role in temporarily arresting cell division when there has been DNA damage (Figure 4.4(a)). This allows time for damage repair prior to subsequent division or if the damage is severe, cell death. It seems probable that some cancers are the result of sublethal damage, which causes chromosomal disorganization and leads to subsequent cell mutation with ultimately tumour development (Figure 4.4(b)). Some tumours have been shown to contain mutations of the p53 gene protein which could therefore have been a primary contributory factor to tumorigenesis. p53 mutations are very common in many tumours but their precise significance is unclear. It is of particular interest that p53 mutations have been described in somatic cells (i.e. all the normal cells in the body) of Li–Fraumeni families and also

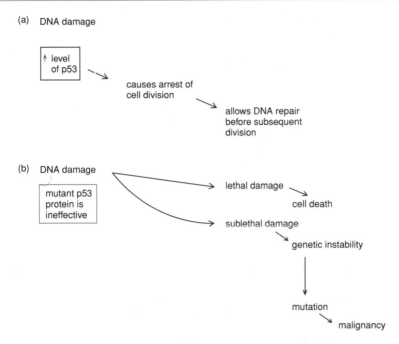

(a)   DNA damage

↑ level
of p53

causes arrest of
cell division

allows DNA repair
before subsequent
division

(b)   DNA damage

mutant p53
protein is
ineffective

lethal damage

cell death

sublethal damage

genetic instability

mutation

malignancy

Figure 4.4 (a) Normal activity of p53 gene product in assisting cell repair. With mutant p53 (b) sublethal damage may fail to be repaired and lead to carcinogenesis.

other familial breast cancer patients. Screening programmes looking for the presence of somatic p53 mutations may lead to the early detection of cancer-prone families with all the ethical and practical implications this would carry. It is difficult to envisage what advice could be given to a family in whom there is a significantly increased risk of rhabdomyosarcoma in a child. Regular CT scanning looking for a small tumour at any of multiple sites is clearly impracticable. Would this information simply lead to anxiety which cannot be readily alleviated?

REFERENCES

Alexander, F., Cartwright, R., McKinney, P.A. and Ricketts, T.J. (1990) Investigation of special clustering of rare diseases: childhood malignancies in North Humberside. *Journal of Epidemiology and Community Health*, **44**, 39–46.

Cartwright, R.A. (1989) Low frequency alternating magnetic fields and leukaemia: the saga so far. *British Journal of Cancer*, **60**, 649–651.

Davis, M.K., Savitz, D.A. and Graubard, B.I. (1988) Infant feeding and childhood cancer. *Lancet*, **ii**, 365–368.

Gardner, M.J., Hall, A.J., Downes, S. and Terrell, J.D. (1987) Follow up study of children born to mothers resident in Seascale, West Cumbria (birth cohort). *British Medical Journal*, **295**, 822–827.

Gardner, M.J., Snee, M.P., Hall, A.J. *et al.* (1990) Results of case-control study of leukaemia and lymphoma among young people near Sellafield nuclear plant in West Cumbria. *British Medical Journal*, **300**, 423–429.

Greaves, M.F. (1988) Speculations on the cause of childhood acute lymphoblastic leukemia. *Leukemia*, **2**, 120–125.

Greaves, M.F. and Chan, L.C. (1986) Is spontaneous mutation the major 'cause' of childhood acute lymphoblastic leukaemia? *British Journal of Haematology*, **64**, 1–13.

Henshaw, D.L., Eatough, J.P. and Richardson, R.B. (1990) Radon as a causative factor in induction of myeloid leukaemia and other cancers. *Lancet*, **335**, 1008–1012.

Israel, M.A. (1992) Molecular biology of pediatric tumors, in *Clinical Applications of Molecular Biology in Cancer* (ed. S. Broder), Williams & Wilkins, Maryland, pp. 267–294.

Kinlen, L. (1990) Evidence for an infective cause of childhood leukaemia: comparison of a Scottish New Town with nuclear reprocessing sites in Britain. *Lancet*, **ii**, 1323–1327.

Lane, D.P. (1992) p53, guardian of the genome. *Nature (London)*, **358**, 15–16.

Levine, E.G., King, R.A. and Bloomfield, C.D. (1989) The role of heredity in cancer. *Journal of Clinical Oncology*, **7**, 527–540.

Li, F.P. and Fraumeni, J.F. (1969) Rhabdomyosarcoma in children: epidemiologic study and identification of a familial cancer syndrome. *Journal of the National Cancer Institute*, **43**, 1365–1373.

Penn, I. (1990) Cancer complicating organ transplantation. *New England Journal of Medicine*, **323**, 1767–1768.

Ponder, B.A.J. (1991) Genetic predisposition to cancer. *British Journal of Cancer*, **64**, 203–204.

Preston-Martin, S., Yu, M.C., Benton, B. and Henderson, B.E. (1982) N-nitroso compounds and childhood brain tumours: a case-control study. *Cancer Research*, **42**, 5240–5245.

Ron, E., Modan, B., Boice, J.D. *et al.* (1988) Tumors of the brain and nervous system after radiotherapy in childhood. *New England Journal of Medicine*, **319**, 1033–1039.

Shu, X.O., Gao, Y.T., Brinton, L.A. *et al.* (1988) A population-based case-control study of childhood leukemia in Shanghai. *Cancer*, **62**, 635–644.

Stiller, C.A. (1991) Aetiology and epidemiology, in *Paediatric Oncology, Clinical Practice and Controversies* (eds P.N. Plowman and C.R. Pinkerton). Chapman & Hall Medical, London, pp. 1–24.

Stiller, C.A., McKinney, P.A., Bunch, K.A. *et al.* (1991) Childhood cancer and ethnic group in Britain: A United Kingdom Children's Cancer Study Group (UKCCSG) Study. *British Journal of Cancer*, **64**, 543–548.

Swinnen, L.J., Costanzo-Nordin, M.R., Fisher, S.G. *et al.* (1990) Increased incidence of lymphoproliferative disorder after immunosuppression with the monoclonal antibody OKT3 in cardiac-transplant recipients. *New England Journal of Medicine*, **323**, 1723–1728.

Weinberg, R.A. (1989) Oncogenes, antioncogenes, and the molecular bases of multistep carcinogenesis. *Cancer Research*, **49**, 3713–3721.

5 | Coping with the diagnosis of cancer

Confirming the diagnosis of cancer to a child's parents is a necessary but unenviable task. The way information about a life-threatening illness is given can affect the parents' ability to come to terms with the diagnosis and if done inappropriately can cause additional unnecessary stress (Woolley *et al.*, 1989). The diagnosis of cancer has an immediate and lasting impact on the family. All members will be affected and can experience feelings of loss of control and uncertainty about their future (Hersh and Wiener, 1989).

After the diagnosis of cancer is made the family must adjust to the demands of the medical care and adapt to all that this entails in order to ensure an environment that promotes health and coping for all the family members.

Individuals' perception of cancer will be dependent upon their age, education, development, culture, economic status and race. All these variables thus create a unique situation for each child and family. As stated earlier, it is an advantage to be treated in a specialized unit where members of the multidisciplinary team have experience in recognizing and understanding families' reactions and can work together to promote adaptive behaviour within the family.

5.1 IMPACT ON THE PARENTS

The diagnosis of cancer represents an assault on parents' identity and sense of adequacy as guardians (Futterman and Hoffman, 1973). On hearing the confirmation of their child's diagnosis parents generally experience intense feelings of shock, fear, disbelief, anger, guilt, depression, apathy and grief. Acute anxiety, hopelessness and confusion are also common. Feelings of disbelief are normal reactions to any unexpected happening. They allow parents to confront the full implications of the disease and its treatment at their own pace and do not overwhelm their ability to face reality. The parents express concern as to the cause of the illness. They may question themselves – 'are we to blame?' – 'could we have prevented this?' – 'is it something we have done or something we have omitted to do? Cancer doesn't just happen for no reason!' They may feel they are being punished for what they see as previous transgressions, such as smoking during pregnancy. All parents, even if they are not verbalizing expressions of guilt, need reassurance that they are not to blame – they did not cause the disease.

As the feelings of disbelief subside they are often replaced by anger. The anger may be directed at the hospital doctors who have confirmed their worst fears, at their G.P. or local hospital, or at God – 'why us?' or at the disease itself for the disruption and distress it will cause. Anger uses up a great deal of energy and can leave parents feeling exhausted and unable to support others around them. The next stage has been described as that of 'demystification' (Austin, 1990). It is the time when parents actively seek out information about the child's condition and try to regain some control. As parents learn more about the disease and its implications, their feelings of anxiety, guilt and anger begin to lessen and they begin to look at ways of restructuring the family's lifestyle to accommodate the disease and its treatment. This next stage has been defined as one of 'conditional acceptance'.

Reactions to the diagnosis may be further intensified if there is a necessity to commence treatment immediately. Not only do the parents have to come to terms with the fact that their child has cancer but also that they must subject them to frightening treatment modalities.

5.2 IMPACT ON THE CHILD

The child's understanding of any illness is primarily determined by their cognitive development. Therefore the impact of cancer on children will depend upon their age, level of development and previous experience.

The young child has no perception of cancer. Their development at this time is one of self-awareness and differentiation from the mother. It is important to address the continuation of normal growth and development; the infant does not have the ability to understand why separation from a carer occurs, why they are denied basic needs like food and exposed to painful procedures.

The toddler may well regress. The search for autonomy may well seem less desirable when threatened with painful procedures and treatments. This regression may be physiological, refusal to continue toilet training or emotional, refusing to talk, join in games or even failure to display appropriate emotions of anger and/or frustration. The toddler does not perceive the disease as a threat but may view the treatment as a punishment. The young child's immediate concerns revolve around hospitalization, separation and fear of medical procedures (Lansky, List and Ritter-Stirr, 1989).

The school age child, 5–7 years, may react with feelings of anger and frustration. The disease and its treatment will disorganize their recently organized world. Anger may be directed at everyone – throwing toys, hitting and biting family members and members of the health care team. They may also regress physiologically losing their will or ability to carry out newly acquired skills. Behaviour such as thumb sucking or needing a comforter may re-emerge. At this age the child sees things as black or white, good or bad. Because of the disruption it causes the cancer may be perceived as bad and its treatment as a punishment.

The older school age child's concerns are those of separation, abandonment, unfamiliar personnel and environment and threats of bodily harm. Normally they are experiencing a time of increasing independence, autonomy and vulnerability. Children of this age will have experience of illness and therefore may have an awareness of the implications of cancer. Alterations in their body image may make them feel insecure around their peers. They may react with acute anxiety and panic – this may be initial or delayed. The child of this age feels that everything has a cause and a purpose. They may see cancer and its treatment as a punishment. They are likely to ask questions about the cause of their illness, the treatment and side effects. They like to have control by learning the name of their disease and other relevant medical terms.

Adolescents in the transition between childhood and adulthood face very particular problems when diagnosed as having cancer. The diagnosis imposes stresses on the adolescent who is striving to develop independence, identity and a functional role in society (Thompson, 1990). They view the treatment as enforcing dependence, compliance and loss of control.

Adolescence has been divided into three levels (Battista, 1986):

Early (12–15 years), a time of rapid physical growth when they have an increased awareness of their own body image; it is strongly connected to how others see them. They may demonstrate angry and rebellious behaviour to try and gain emotional independence from their family.

Middle adolescence (15–18 years). The time that physical maturity is almost complete. They have a realistic self/body image and are establishing stronger peer group relationships.

Late adolescence (18–22 years). The time concerned with planning future roles and goals and the steps needed to achieve them.

Adolescents possess an increased awareness of cancer and its implications and this can affect their ability to continue their normal daily activities.

They are resentful of the changes that the disease and its treatment will make in their lifestyle. They may become withdrawn and depressed and experience feelings of bitterness and anger.

Fears about alteration in their body image are important as are feelings about physical weakness and vulnerability. These can greatly affect relationships with peers and may prevent them from feeling able to return to school. The implications of the disease and its treatment may affect the long term goals or future plans for the adolescent. They may have to reconsider their career in the light of difficulty in achieving academic requirements or physical disability. These adjustments may cause additional feelings of anger, frustration and jealousy towards their peers. Wherever possible relationships with peers should be encouraged to promote self-esteem and reduce fears of rejection and abandonment. It is important that the adolescent receives constant reassurance that they are the same person that they were before the cancer was diagnosed. Concerns about sexuality must also be addressed. Fertility (sometimes impaired) and impotence (invariable unimpaired) are often confused.

Siblings. The effect on the siblings is again dependent upon their age and level of development and also their age in relation to the ill sibling. Their initial feelings may be those of disbelief that the sibling is very ill and jealousy that their parents have to spend so much time with them.

The causes of stress in children whose sibling has cancer are multiple (Walker, 1988). They include loss of parental attention, identification with the sick sibling, concerns over the change in the family structure, role and activity and worries regarding the cause of the cancer. Experiences of guilt, jealousy, shame and fears about the physical and emotional side effects of the treatment on their sibling have also been described. The parents appear to be preoccupied with the ill child and this limits the amount of support and attention given to the well siblings who feel their lives have been disrupted by the frequent visits and stays in hospital. They may be cared for by members of the extended family or friends while the ill child has sole attention of the parents. The ill child appears to receive preferential treatment – missing days from school, receiving special treats for coping with the demands of the disease of its treatment. The well child may experience difficulties at school facing endless questions about their sibling's condition and perhaps insensitive teasing about alteration in body image or outcome of the disease.

Altered body images such as hair loss, obesity, weight loss, limb amputation can be frightening for siblings to witness and the effects of the disease or the toxicity of its treatment such as febrile neutropenia puzzling and difficult to understand (Kramer and Moore, 1983). All these fears and anxieties affect their ability to cope. They may seek attention by changing their behaviour – regressing physically or emotionally, bed wetting, poor attention at school, emotional outbursts or by throwing themselves into their school work looking for a sense of value and self worth. The parents' ability to cope with these additional stresses is often exhausted and family support appears unavailable. The well child feels neglected, unable to discuss all the worries and fears that they have. Siblings may be reluctant to confront their parents at this time because they feel insecure about their position in the family (Cairns *et al.*, 1979).

5.3 CONFIRMING THE DIAGNOSIS

Parents vividly remember the manner in which the diagnosis of a life-threatening illness is given (Woolley *et al.*, 1989). It is essential, therefore, that the confirmation of cancer to parents should be a planned event. The approach of the hospital team at the time of diagnosis can affect the parents' ability to begin to come to terms with the diagnosis and will also affect the establishment of a collaborative, trustful relationship (Levine, Blumberg and Hersh, 1982).

Interviews with parents should take place in private rooms with no interruptions. Giving information to both parents at the same time prevents one parent having to remember what was said or being responsible for confirming the 'bad news'. It also avoids the risk of parents interpreting the information differently and feeling that the doctor may have told their spouse something extra or different. Being together also facilitates discussion and sharing.

Parents may find it useful to have a nurse present who can reassure and clarify confusing issues. Flexibility as to the amount and level of information given is required, repetition and clarification have also been identified as being beneficial. Openness and sensitivity encourages parents to feel comfortable and encourages them to ask questions. It is beneficial to use direct words such as fear, anger and death as this conveys the ability and willingness to discuss difficult subjects. Phrases such as 'a little worried' should be avoided (Martocchio, 1985). The information given should be truthful and offer positive support but not unrealistic hope. Subsequent meetings should be arranged and suggestions of writing down questions as they occur for discussion at the next meeting may be of use to the parents. Written information to back up the conversation is also very helpful.

Following the meeting parents should also be offered the opportunity to have some time together in private to share their feelings and prepare themselves to face their child. The child needs to be told as much about his disease and its treatment as he is able to understand. The information should be given in language appropriate for his level of development. Parents often find it helpful if the initial details of the disease and treatment are given by medical or nursing staff.

Parents may request that the child is not told the truth in order to protect them. However it is impossible to keep the severity of the illness from the child. The mannerisms of all around him will have indicated that this is not an everyday occurrence. To hide the truth may make the child imagine a much worse illness and outcome. They may compare symptoms with the child in the next bed and guess at the diagnosis, perhaps incorrectly. Confirming the diagnosis may create fear in the child but treating them with secrecy may prevent them from asking important questions. The child may observe that the diagnosis upsets their parents and may try to prevent upsetting them more by not talking about it even though they may have many questions and fears.

Communication between the child and parents about the disease should be encouraged, to avoid increasing fears and anxieties of the child. Family stress can be considerably alleviated once the child understands and accepts the diagnosis and that this paves the way for more open communication within the family (Hersh and Wiener, 1990). It may, indeed, be easier for the children to learn about their illness than the parents because they do not have the same preconceptions about cancer.

5.4 PREPARATION FOR TREATMENT

Preparation for treatment includes the psychological preparation as well as the physical. Before sharing information with the child it is important to assess the knowledge or perception that the child already has. This will assist in recognizing the child's needs and facilitate a structured sharing of information. Children's fantasies may help or hinder their ability to develop new coping strategies and it has been stated that 'a child's defences should not be broken down unless one is sure that more desirable concepts will take their place' (Blatti, 1985). Fantasy in children may be comparable to the denial that parents display, providing them with time to come to terms with their diagnosis or aspects of their treatment and its side effects. Forcing a child to face things before they are ready may be counter-productive. The type, level and amount of information about the specific treatment will also depend upon the age and level of development of the patient. Issues related to altered body image or body function should be addressed with sensitivity and whenever possible time for adjustment to come to terms with the information should be allowed.

Verbal information may be backed up with written information, again providing the patient with the opportunity to clarify issues.

The play therapist and psychologist/psychiatrist have an important role in assessing the coping and adaptive mechanisms displayed by the patient and helping them appropriately.

The physical preparation will depend upon the specific treatment and will be discussed in the different treatment modality chapters. If a central line has not already been inserted, it is likely to be required now.

Gaining knowledge about the disease, treatment and side effects enables the children to feel they have some control and helps them to come to terms more easily. Studies with adolescents indicated they required simple understandable explanations with reassurance about possible outcomes (Orr, Hoffmans and Bennetts, 1984). Accurate and honest information facilitates establishment of trusting relationships. Encouraging active participation in decision making about treatment plans, including its timing, enables them to have choice and a degree of flexibility helps toward a feeling of control and independence.

Adolescent units facilitate the camaraderie and acceptance of peers and offer the opportunity of discussing with peers the effects of the disease and treatments. When adolescent units are not available paediatric units are probably preferable to adult cancer units as there is greater emphasis on the psychosocial and developmental needs of the patient and family (Lansky, List and Ritter-Stirr, 1989).

If the siblings are to cope and survive emotionally they need to understand and be involved in the care of their sick brother or sister. Showing an interest in the siblings – getting to know them by name and involving them assist in making them feel part of the team. Sharing knowledge about the disease, its treatment, side effects and implications for them, such as time to be spent in hospital, are important to help the well sibling adjust to the disorganization of his family life. The well siblings require appropriate preparation for the physical and emotional changes the ill child may have. Parents need encouragement and support to meet the needs of their healthy child as well as coping with the demands of the sick one. The degree of communication between parents and siblings has been shown to influence how well the siblings coped (Spinetta and Deasy-Spinetta, 1981).

5.5 COPING MECHANISMS

The stress that families experience following the diagnosis of cancer will be unlike any other encountered in their daily lives. The development and recognition of coping strategies for the family is therefore vital. The goal for all members of the health care team is to help the family integrate the fact of the disease, its treatment and the side effects into the family life. Families experience feelings of entering a crisis situation at the time of diagnosis. Crisis has been defined as an insoluble problem brought on by stressful events, causing loss of equilibrium in an individual (Lewis, Gottesman and Gutstein, 1979). A crisis is usually limited to 4–6 weeks and it motivates the development of coping mechanisms, which in turn may be useful in solving future stresses. The crisis will resolve only when effective coping mechanisms are established.

The return to a state of equilibrium in the family or individual is dependent on adaptive coping. Coping involves regaining control and mastering the situation; it is a process to resolve a stressful situation. It does not imply an absence of problems. Factors that influence families' abilities to develop new coping strategies include the behaviour and belief of the family members, previous experience with stressful situations, individuals' coping strategies, the family dynamics and the socio-economic background.

In many families the role of the health care team will be that of supporter, educator and facilitator. Family members need support and encouragement to discuss their concerns and worries. The appropriate members of the health care team can facilitate communication between family members, helping them to share problems and discuss possible solutions.

Information about members of the family, how they interact with each other, their individual roles and previous experience with stressful situations enables the members of the health care team to assess the impact of the disease and suggest plans to help the family identify problems and means of dealing with them. As mentioned previously, parents who have difficulty coming to terms with their child's diagnosis and the implications that the treatment may have, physically and emotionally, for the child and financially for the family, may neglect their own and their family's care. Encouraging parents to talk about the family may therefore help them to look at the needs of all of the family. It must not be assumed that all family members will experience the same stresses. Each individual may face multiple stresses, some of which may be unique. However, families benefit from being informed that their own responses are understandable and appropriate (Lansky, List and Ritter-Stirr, 1989).

As previously mentioned, coping involves regaining control or mastering the situation. To enable families to do this they need information about the disease, the treatment and side effects. The information should be given both verbally and in writing and repeated as frequently as the parents, siblings or patient requires. Information about self-help groups and community support is also of value.

Two factors that affect families' coping ability are firstly their experience in coping as a supportive team and secondly their ability to participate in the child's care (Martocchio, 1985). If the family are not able to gain support from each other they may look to outsiders to help their child; equally if they do not feel able to participate in the care of their child but observe 'strangers' caring they may experience feelings of loss of control and helplessness. Recognizing and encouraging the knowledge and skills that the parents have about their child makes them feel a valuable member of the team.

The following points have been described as essential coping tasks for parents (Hockenberry, 1986):

1. gaining control of their emotions by having time and space to grieve;
2. alleviating their acute anxieties by encouraging the expression of their feelings and fears and encouraging the maintenance of hope;
3. developing an understanding of the diagnosis by information sharing and discussion;
4. enabling the parents to explain the diagnosis to their child by identifying the rational and providing the information and support;
5. establishing the treatment, with education of the parents about the methods of administration, the side effects and their participation;
6. preventing anxieties about discharge and care at home by early discussion about the return to home and identifying key people to help;
7. participation of other family members by discussion with them about the treatment and side effects and encouraging them to visit and participate in the child's care.

Five psychological issues have been identified as being important for adolescents with cancer to master to enable them to cope effectively (Blotcky, 1986). These are: (i) maintenance of normal development, (ii) an understanding of the disease, (iii) tolerance of painful or invasive procedures, (iv) control of behavioral side effects of the therapy, and (v) family issues.

Working with the adolescent and their family and focusing on existing coping strategies enables the adolescent to perceive the disease and treatment as manageable and provides a feeling of optimism and hope. As the adolescent and family's advocate, the nurse works with them to achieve a level of adjustment that is acceptable and that they are able to maintain. It has been suggested that it is helpful for adolescents to practise how they will respond to certain situations that may occur once discharged from hospital prior to their discharge (Battista, 1986).

Encouragement to return to school may be reassuring in relation to the success of the treatment and emphasizes the importance of setting goals. Factors that affect a child's ability to cope include the child/parent relationship, the age of the child and level of development, the family's acceptance of the disease and previously developed coping strategies.

Facilitating adjustment by the patients and siblings requires: (i) participation in the particular family system, (ii) providing information about disease, treatment and side effects, (iii) continued interaction with the parents, and (iv) encouraging their participation in the care of the ill sibling, and (v) developing an understanding of the illness and its complications on the family unit.

Coping with the crisis of cancer requires the development of new attitudes, behaviours and coping techniques (Van Eys, 1977). The health care team are facilitators to enable the family to develop a way of life that is acceptable and comparable to the one before the diagnosis, whilst complying with the treatment and all its implications.

REFERENCES

Austin, J. (1990) Assessment of coping mechanisms used by parents and children with chronic illness. *American Journal of Maternal and Child Nursing*, **15**, 98–102.

Battista, E. (1986) Educational needs of the adolescent with cancer and his family. *Seminars in Oncology Nursing*, **2**(2), 123–125.

Blatti, G. (1985) Developmental aspects of chronic illness: Cancer in the childhood years. *Cancer Nursing* Suppl. 17–20.

Blotcky, A. (1986) Helping adolescents with cancer cope with their disease. *Seminars in Oncology Nursing*, **2**(2), 117–122.

Cairns, N.U., Clark, G.M., Smith, S.D. and Lansky, S.B. (1979) Adaptation of siblings to childhood malignancies. *Journal of Paediatrics*, **995**, 484–487.

Futterman, E.H. and Hoffman, I. (1973) Crisis adaptation in the families of fatally ill children, in *The Child and His Family* (eds E.J. Anthony and E. Koipernik) Wiley & Sons, New York, 127–143.

Hersh, S.P. and Wiener, L.S. (1990) Psychosocial support for the family of the child with cancer, in *Principles and Practice of Paediatric Oncology* (eds P.A. Pizzo and D.G. Poplack) **42**, 897–913.

Hockenberry, M. (1986) Crisis point in cancer, in *Paediatric Oncology and Haematology – Perspectives on Care* (eds M. Hockenberry and D. Coody) C.V. Mosby, St. Louis, 432–449.

Kendrick, C., Culling, S., Oakhill, T. *et al.* Children's understanding of their illness and its treatment within a paediatric oncology unit. (Unpublished article.)

Kramer, R.F. and Moore, I.M. (1983) Childhood cancer – meeting the special needs of healthy siblings. *Cancer Nursing*, **6**, 213–217.

Lansky, S.B., List, M.A. and Ritter-Stirr, C. (1989) Psychiatric and psychological support of the child and adolescent with cancer, in *Principles and Practice of Paediatric Oncology* (eds P.A. Pizzo and D.G. Poplack) Lippincott, Philadelphia.

Levine, A.S., Blumberg, B.D. and Hersh, S.P. (1982) The psychosocial concomitants of cancer in young patients, in *Cancer in the Young* (ed. A.S. Levine) Masson, New York, USA.

Lewis, M.S., Gottesman, D. and Gutstein, S. (1979) The cause and duration of crisis. *Journal of Consulting and Clinical Psychology*, **47**(1), 128–131.

Martocchio, B. (1985) Family coping – helping families to help themselves. *Seminars in Oncology Nursing*, **1**(4), 292–297.

Orr, D.P., Hoffmans, M.A. and Bennetts, G. (1984) Adolescents with cancer report their psychosocial needs. *Journal of Psychosocial Oncology*, **2**(2), 47–59.

Spinetta, J. and Deasy-Spinetta, P. (1981) *Living with Childhood Cancer*, C.V. Mosby, St Louis.

Thompson, J. (1990) The adolescent with cancer, in *The Child with Cancer – Nursing Care*, Scutari, London, pp. 127–139.

Van Eys, J. (1977) *The Truly Cured Child*. University Park Press, Baltimore.

Walker, C. (1988) Stress and coping in siblings of childhood cancer patients. *Nursing Research*, **37**(4), 208–212.

Woolley, H., Stein, A. and Forrest, G.C. (1989) Imparting the diagnosis of life threatening illness in children. *British Medical Journal*, **298**, 1623–1626.

Chemotherapy

6

6.1 INTRODUCTION

The term chemotherapy refers to the use of cytotoxic agents, i.e. drugs toxic to cells. These interfere with the proliferation of cells and are an effective and often curative method of treatment for many types of tumour and leukaemia. Chemotherapy drugs are administered singly or in combination. The drugs may be used as the sole treatment modality or in combination with surgery and/or radiotherapy.

Although medical staff prescribe cytotoxic therapy, it is increasingly becoming the responsibility of the specialist nurse to administer the drug. Consequently a sound knowledge is required of:

1. The mechanisms of cytotoxic agents.
2. Their safe administration to the patient and for the nurse.
3. Immediate, short and long term side effects.

The nurse should ultimately be able to deliver safe care, detect any adverse side effects and educate the parents and children appropriately.

6.2 CELL CYCLE

Knowledge of the nature of the cell cycle is necessary to understand the action of the cytotoxic therapy. G_0 is the inactive phase when no division takes place (Figure 6.1). The cycle begins with the G_1 and 'S' phases. During this phase the cell manufactures DNA prior to DNA replication. During 'S' phase the DNA content of the cell is doubled so that when the cell passes to the mitotic 'M' phase two daughter cells, identical to the parent cell are produced.

The percentage of tumour cells in the G_0 phase may be a significant factor of tumour relapse. If the cells are in the inactive resting phase, cell cycle specific cytotoxic drugs are unable to affect them and primary

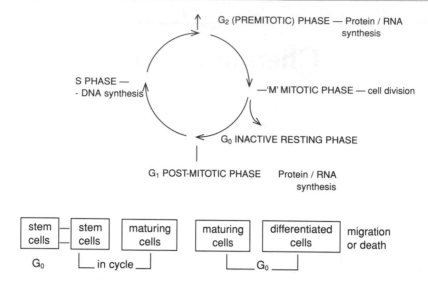

Figure 6.1 Cell and maturation cycles.

resistance or regrowth of tumour may occur. A tumour with a high 'growth fraction', i.e. in cycle, will be more chemosensitive.

Cancer cells may deviate from the normal cell cycle, dividing into more than two daughter cells during mitosis of the cell cycle or resulting in grossly abnormal chromosome structures. They also appear to fail to recognize the growth inhibiting factors recognized by normal cells. Figure 6.1 also shows the normal evolution from a resting stem cell, through the active cycling phase to a second resting phase, during which functional and structural maturation occurs.

The cells of the bone marrow and the gastrointestinal tract are continually proliferating and thus it is these tissues which are commonly adversely affected by cytotoxic therapy. The toxic effects of chemotherapy on these two tissues may be a major limiting factor in the tolerance of chemotherapy.

Chemotherapeutic drugs can be broadly divided into three categories (Figure 6.2):

1. The cell cycle specific drugs which affect the cycle during specific phases, e.g. the 'M' or the 'S' phase.
2. The cell cycle non-specific drugs which affect the cycle during *all* phases of the cell cycle.
3. Less commonly – non-cell cycle specific.

The aim of chemotherapy is to destroy all the cancer cells, therefore it is usual to administer a combination of cell cycle specific and cell cycle non-specific drugs for potential optimum affect.

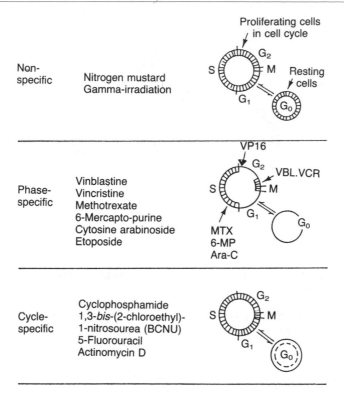

Figure 6.2 Phases of cell cycle in dividing cell. The sites of action of phase- and cycle-specific agents are listed.

6.3 CHEMOTHERAPY DRUGS

Antimetabolites

This group of drugs resembles natural compounds involved in cell replication. These compete with or block the natural compound.

Methotrexate (MTX)

The synthesis of purine nucleotides, thymidylate and the amino acids serine and methionine is dependent on the presence of reduced folates, i.e. tetrahydrofolates (FH4).

Dihydrofolate reductase (DHFR) is the enzyme responsible for maintaining the level of intracellular FH4. Methotrexate resembles folic acid (Figure 6.3) and is a potent inhibitor of DHFR. This causes an accumulation of folate in the inactive oxidized form, with consequent cell death.

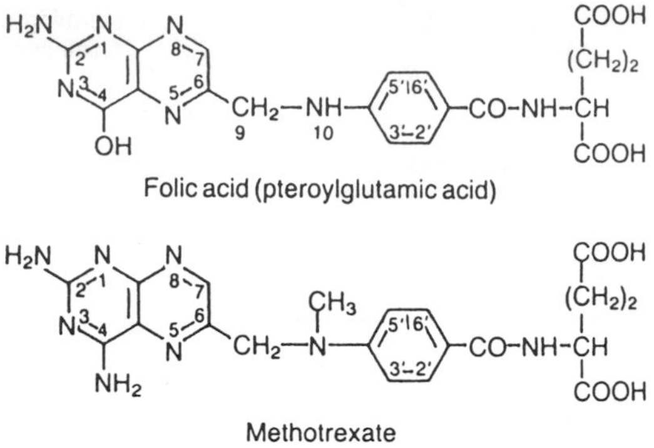

Folic acid (pteroylglutamic acid)

Methotrexate

Figure 6.3 Comparative structure of folic acid and the antagonist methotrexate showing the close homology.

There are a number of different mechanisms by which tumour cells can develop resistance to MTX:

1. Amplification of the DHFR gene results in increased levels of intracellular DHFR, thus overcoming the MTX inhibition of the enzyme.
2. The affinity of DHFR for MTX can be reduced by minor alterations in the structure of the enzyme.
3. Impaired transport of MTX into the cell.

Administration of folinic acid 24–36 hours after methotrexate bypasses the latter's site of action and allows normal cell division. This enables very high doses of methotrexate to be given safely provided adequate 'rescue' is given. Serum methotrexate levels must be carefully monitored so that the dose of folinic acid can be increased or rescue prolonged. This strategy is used in ALL and non-Hodgkin's lymphoma in order to increase central nervous system drug penetration (Figure 6.4). In osteosarcoma this approach increases tumour tissue drug levels.

5-Fluorouracil (5-FU)

This drug requires intracellular conversion to its active components, which include fluorouridine triphosphate (FUTP) and 5-fluorodeoxyuridylate (5-FdUMP). The former is incorporated into nuclear RNA and inhibits RNA processing and function. The latter binds to the enzyme thymidylate synthase (TS) thus inhibiting the formation of deoxythymidine triphosphate (dTTP) an essential precursor of DNA. Resistance can develop following depletion of the enzymes required for 5-FU activation or following amplification of the (TS) gene resulting in increased levels of the enzyme.

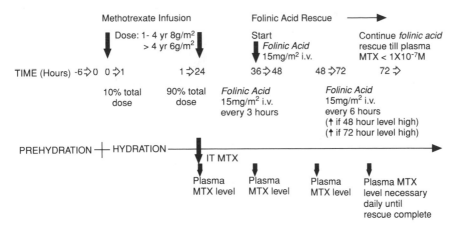

Figure 6.4 Schema of high dose methotrexate/folinic acid rescue in ALL.

Cytarabine

Cytarabine (cytosine arabinoside, Ara-C) is structurally very similar to the naturally occurring cytidine nucleoside, deoxycytidine. It is metabolized inside the cell to its active form, Ara-CTP, and competes with deoxycytidine triphosphate (dCTP) thus inhibiting DNA polymerase and interfering with DNA replication (Figure 6.5). It is also incorporated into DNA and interferes with DNA transcription.

Mechanisms of resistance to cytarabine include the depletion of activating enzymes, an increase in the intracellular pool of dCTP and increased ability of tumour cells to eliminate Ara-CTP.

6-Mercaptopurine (6-MP) and 6-Thioguanine (6-TG)

These closely resemble the purine nucleosides hypoxanthine and guanine. Following intracellular activation by their conversion to 'fraudulent' nucleotides they are incorporated into DNA and result in faulty DNA replication and the development of strand breaks, the frequency of which is correlated with toxicity.

6-MP resistant cells lack the activating enzyme hypoxanthine-guanine phosphoribosyl transferase (HGPRTase) (Figure 6.6). Thiopurine methyltransferase (TPMT) metabolises 6-MP to an inactive form. Some patients, especially males, have higher TPMT levels and consequently the number of cytotoxic 6-TG nucleotides is reduced. In contrast, very low levels of TPMT will be associated with poor tolerance of 6-MP.

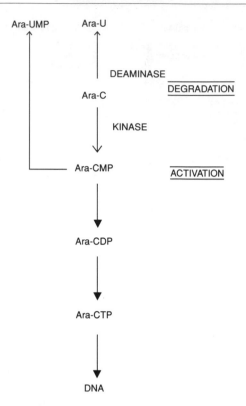

Figure 6.5 Metabolism of cytarabine (Ara-C). Both Ara-C and its metabolite deoxycytosine monophosphate (Ara-CMP) are inactivated by deaminase. A series of kinase enzymes metabolizes Ara-C through the monophosphate (Ara-CMP), and diphosphate (Ara-CDP) compounds to the active triphosphate metabolite (Ara-CTP).

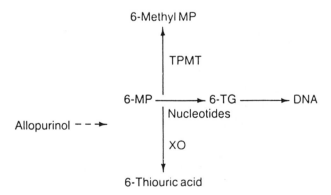

Figure 6.6 Metabolism of 6-mercaptopurine (6-MP) to either the active 6-thioguanine nucleotides (6-TG) or the inactive 6-methyl mercaptopurine (6-methyl MP) and 6-thiouric acid. Allopurinol blocks xanthine oxidase (XO) and will increase toxicity.

Alkylating agents

Nitrogen mustard was the first cytotoxic agent to come into clinical use but is now rarely used because of toxicity. Cyclophosphamide and its analogue ifosfamide are active against a wide range of solid and haematological malignancies. Both these agents are metabolized to their active forms (Figure 6.7). Ifosfamide is less myelosuppressive than cyclophosphamide and consequently higher doses can be given. Unfortunately it is toxic to the renal tubules particularly in young children and high doses of cyclophosphamide, using bone marrow growth factors, may be equally effective. Other commonly used alkylating agents include chlorambucil, melphalan and busulphan.

The cytotoxicity of the alkylating agents is thought to relate to their ability to form covalent bonds with bases in DNA. It is not fully understood how the process of alkylation results in cytotoxicity but it is thought that the cross-linking and strand breaks in DNA that develop following exposure of cells to these agents interferes with the integrity of DNA causing misreading of the DNA code and inhibition of DNA, RNA and protein synthesis.

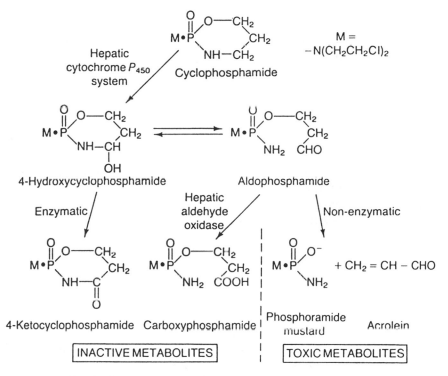

Figure 6.7 Metabolism of cyclophosphamide to its inactive metabolites, the cytotoxic mustard derivative and the bladder-toxic acrolein.

The activity of alkylating agents within cells can be inhibited by conjugation to glutathione (GSH) and high levels of GSH in tumour may correlate with drug resistance. Another mechanism of resistance involves the rapid repair of DNA damage by DNA repair enzymes.

Nitrosoureas

The nitrosoureas CCNU and BCNU are generally classed as alkylating agents, but differ somewhat in their mode of action. In aqueous solution they are broken down into two reactive intermediates. The first binds to a single strand of DNA producing a second reactive site that results in DNA cross-linking. The second is thought to deplete glutathione, inhibit DNA repair and interfere with RNA. These agents do not share cross-resistance with the classical alkylators. Although resistance can be similarly attributed to increased levels of GSH and DNA repair enzymes. This group of drugs is rarely used in paediatrics because of their association with induction of secondary leukaemia. The exception is in brain tumours where excellent CNS penetration is achieved.

Platinum compounds

Cis (II) platinum diamminedichloride (cisplatin) is a tetravalent heavy metal compound with two chloride ions bound to two amine groups.

$$NH_3 \diagdown \quad Cl$$
$$Pt$$
$$NH_3 \diagup \quad Cl$$

Cisplatin can react with DNA only after at least one chloride ligand is replaced by water. This occurs most readily in an environment of low chloride concentration, e.g. intracellularly or in urine. Following the replacement of both chloride groups a diaquo form is produced which forms both intra- and interstrand cross links as seen with the alkylators. The cytotoxicity of cisplatin has been correlated with the formation of DNA interstrand cross links, changes in DNA conformation and inhibition of DNA synthesis.

Platinum compounds do not share cross-resistance with the classic alkylating agents or nitrosoureas. Some platinum resistant cell lines have been shown to form DNA cross links at a reduced rate, suggesting either slower drug uptake, impaired activation or rapid repair of DNA damage. Carboplatin (cis-diammino-1,1-cyclobutanedicarboxylatoplatinum (II)) is an analogue of cisplatin which is structurally related but has a bidentate dicarboxylate chelate ligand replacing the two chlorine atoms.

$$NH_3 \diagdown \quad O\!-\!CO \quad CH_2$$

This drug has been shown to be as effective as cisplatin in several tumour types but is considerably less toxic although more myelosuppressive. The dose limiting effects with cisplatin are reduced glomerular filtration rate and high tone hearing loss. These are of obvious importance in children with curable tumours. Continuous infusion of cisplatin over 3–5 days appears to reduce toxicity. The two compounds appear to have the same mechanism of action and differ only in the kinetics of their interaction with DNA.

Vinca alkaloids

The vinca alkaloids (vincristine, vinblastine and vindesine) are natural products derived from the plant *Vinca rosea*. Their mechanism of action relates to their ability to bind to tubulin. This protein is found in the cytoplasm of all cells and is important for maintaining the cytoskeleton and for the formation of the mitotic spindle along which chromosomes migrate during mitosis. The alkaloids thus interfere with the function of the mitotic spindle during cell division and arrest cells in the metaphase of mitosis. The vinca–tubulin complex appears to be more stable in tumour tissue compared to normal tissues which may contribute some selectivity towards malignant cells.

Mutations in tubular structure can result in altered drug binding and lead to drug resistance. When given in a weekly schedule vincristine may cause severe constipation and even paralytic ileus. Regular laxatives such as lactulose are advisable. Peripheral neurotoxicity with loss of ankle and knee reflexes is not uncommon and if weakness occurs the drug is discontinued. This is invariably reversible. Vinblastine is less neurotoxic but unlike vincristine causes myelosuppression. The primary mechanism of resistance to the vinca alkaloids is probably due to decreased intracellular drug accumulation. This results from the increased efflux of drug secondary to the over-expression of a gene that codes for a P-glycoprotein efflux pump found in the cell membrane.

This is the mechanism of multidrug resistance (MDR) whereby tumour cells are resistant to several structurally unrelated drugs without necessarily having been exposed to them. These include daunorubicin, doxorubicin, etoposide, vincristine and amsacrine.

The gene coding for the P-glycoprotein pump (MDR_1 gene) has been shown to be over-expressed in certain multidrug resistant cell lines and tumours. Various drugs can reverse MDR *in vitro*, including the calcium channel blockers verapamil, nifedipine and perhexilene and the calmodulin inhibitors (perfenazine and cyclosporin A). Several clinical trials are currently being undertaken to determine whether these agents might effectively overcome resistance *in vivo*.

Epipodophyllotoxins

The two commonly used epipodophyllotoxins, etoposide (VP-16) and teniposide (VM-26), are synthetic derivatives of podophyllotoxin, an extract from the mandrake plant. The principal target of both etoposide and teniposide is cellular DNA and involves the nuclear enzyme topoisomerase II. Unwinding of the DNA helix during replication and transcription is facilitated by controlled cleavage of the strands (Figure 6.8). The enzyme forms a bridge across the double-stranded DNA break which allows passage of the complementary strand. Topoisomerase inhibitors stabilize the DNA/protein 'cleavable complex' so that the normally rapid processes of strand division, strand passing and rejoining are arrested.

Resistance to the epipodophyllotoxins is multifactorial. Possible mechanisms include:

1. Decreased formation of topoisomerase II induced strand breaks secondary to changes in the amount of the enzyme present or its ability to function following mutational change.
2. Increased repair of DNA strand breaks.
3. Decreased drug accumulation secondary to increased drug efflux due to amplification of the MDR exit pump.

Antitumour antibiotics

These compounds were originally derived from bacteria and fungi and have both antimicrobial and antitumour activity. Subsequently, a number of analogues have been synthesized. The group therefore consists of a diverse range of drugs which differ in structure and mechanisms of action.

Anthracyclines

Daunorubicin and doxorubicin are the anthracyclines most commonly used in clinical practice. Epirubicin (4′-epidoxorubicin) is structurally very similar and the best known of the many anthracycline analogues.

These compounds have a characteristic structure consisting of a planar anthracycline ring attached to an amino sugar. The planar ring allows the molecule to intercalate DNA, i.e. to insert itself within the DNA helix. There is considerable debate about the primary mechanism of action of these drugs. It is possible that there are multiple mechanisms of cell kill and that in any one tumour cell line or tissue, one or other mechanism may predominate. There is good evidence that interference with topo-

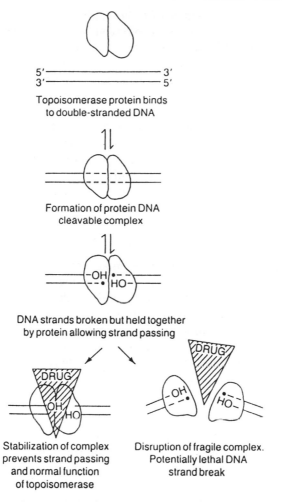

Figure 6.8 Schematic representation of the action of topoisomerase II and the effect of drugs such as etoposide on its function.

isomerase II is responsible for the antitumour activity in some cell lines but the formation of free radicals is probably equally important. This mechanism involves the reduction of molecular oxygen to superoxide and/or hydrogen peroxide. These in turn can react via a variety of mechanisms to yield a hydroxyl radical that causes direct tissue injury. It has been shown in a number of cell systems that iron must be present for anthracycline free-radical formation to result in significant damage. This is also the mechanism of the main toxicity of this group of drugs, namely cardiotoxicity. In the past cumulative doses up to 350–400 mg/m^2 were regarded as safe. Above this the risk of cardiac failure was greater than 10%. Recently detailed echocardiography studies have demonstrated abnormalities at lower doses. Prolonged infusion schedules are less cardiotoxic and rapid bolus infusions should be avoided.

Tumour tissue with *in vitro* resistance to doxorubicin has been shown to express P-glycoprotein whereas only a small number of P-glycoprotein-negative tumours were resistant. Several experimental systems such as these have implicated the role of the MDR mechanism in clinical resistance to anthracyclines. Enhanced neutralization of anthracycline-induced free radicals by the glutathione redox system may also be involved.

Mitozantrone is a synthetic compound classed as an anthracedione and is a hydroxyquinone with a similar ring structure to the anthracyclines. It does not, however, cause free-radical damage but does induce topoisomerase-II-mediated DNA damage.

Bleomycin

Bleomycin is a mixture of low molecular weight glycopeptides derived from a fungus. Its cytotoxicity results from the ability to bind to and degrade DNA. Lung toxicity, particularly with weekly schedules, has reduced the use of this drug in children. Anaesthesia with oxygen may exacerbate lung toxicity and should be avoided, e.g. repeated CT scans in infants. Resistance can be related to enhanced DNA repair. Similarly, intracellular bleomycin-inactivating enzymes may be important determinants of tumour cell sensitivity.

Actinomycin D

This drug consists of two identical cyclic polypeptides bound to a phenoxazone ring. Following intercalation of the ring structure into the DNA double helix the polypeptide chains block both DNA and RNA synthesis. Actinomycin D can also form single-strand breaks following reduction of the molecule to radical intermediates or via topoisomerase II. The relevance of these strand breaks to the cytotoxicity of the drug is not, however, totally clear.

Both actinomycin and the anthracyclines can potentiate radiation toxicity and are avoided during radiotherapy. Radiation 'recall' can occur when these drugs follow irradiation resulting in skin erythema and desquamation in some cases.

Miscellaneous agents

Dacarbazine (DTIC)

Dacarbazine is a synthetic compound found by chance to have antimitotic activity. It functions as an alkylating agent following metabolic activation to an active species. In addition, one of the metabolites formed in the process inhibits the incorporation of purine nucleosides into DNA.

Procarbazine

Procarbazine was discovered during a search for new monoamine oxidase inhibitors. Its exact mechanism of action is not completely understood although it is likely to involve alkylation following microsomal metabolic activation.

Amsacrine (mAMSA)

Amsacrine (mAMSA) was one of the first agents whose mechanism of action was shown to involve topoisomerase. It forms a tight complex with DNA and topoisomerase II and prevents the resealing of DNA breaks. The cytotoxicity of the drug correlates closely with the production of both single- and double-strand DNA breaks. Drug resistance appears related to altered topoisomerase II, which no longer cleaves DNA in the presence of amsacrine.

L-Asparaginase

This drug has a unique tumour-specific mechanism of action. L-asparagine is a non-essential amino acid synthesized by the transamination of L-aspartic acid by L-asparagine synthetase. Certain malignant cells are unable to synthesize asparagine and rely on the body pool for the supply of this amino acid. L-asparaginase converts asparagine to aspartic acid and ammonia thus depriving tumour cells of an essential nutrient. Its antitumour effect is therefore related to the depletion of circulating pools of L-asparagine whereas resistance is related to an increase in L-asparagine synthetase activity following either mutation or enzyme induction.

Pancreatitis is an unusual complication with this drug and serum amylase levels should be checked if abdominal pain develops during its use. Coagulation defects may rarely develop due to an effect on liver function.

Hydroxyurea

Hydroxyurea is an analogue of urea. It acts by inhibiting the ribonucleotide reductase enzyme system, thereby preventing DNA synthesis. It is one of the few specific S phase inhibitors.

Corticosteroids

Steroid therapy is used for symptom relief, e.g. the management of raised intracranial pressure and bone pain. There is also a direct antitumour effect, particularly in haematological malignancies, by mechanisms that are not clearly understood but which may involve glucocorticoid receptors on the tumour cell.

6.4 ADMINISTRATION OF CHEMOTHERAPY

Safe handling of cytotoxic drugs has become a topic of great debate with emphasis on those administering them. There have been a number of studies to determine whether cytotoxic agents are absorbed by the administrator. In one study (Ames *et al.*, 1975), whilst urinalysis was positive, the analytical methods have been questioned and the long term effects of the findings inconclusive. However, the fundamental issue of developing precautionary methods to prevent any absorption of cytotoxic agents remains uncontested.

Protective methods during the handling and administration of cytotoxic drugs may vary between units and therefore those concerned should refer to local policy, for which guidelines should be readily available. Adequate staff training clearly plays a vital role.

Increasingly, the reconstitution of drugs is carried out by technicians in specialised areas with laminar air flow facilities. Although the nature of protective clothing may vary, most units recommend goggles, gloves, gowns or aprons, and also masks when dealing with powdered drugs.

Having established safety needs for the individual who administers the chemotherapy, patient safety becomes the next priority. The administration of cytotoxic therapy without ensuring that all the pre-chemotherapy tests have been completed and the results available, can lead to dangerous toxicity and, in the extreme, be fatal. Both the nurse and doctor should be responsible for checking the baseline results.

Investigations required prior to therapy will be individual to each protocol and should be clearly documented with easy access to nurses/ doctors in the unit. Examples of baseline investigations are listed below:

Full blood count with differential
Urea, electrolytes and liver
    function test   } Instructions as to when to delay
Kidney function test   therapy or dose adjust is
                                 individual to each protocol
Height and weight
General health of child   Bone marrow aspiration
Condition of mouth   Lumbar puncture
                           Chest X-ray

Temperature, pulse and blood pressure

Staging investigation – ultrasound
– CT scan

Of equal importance to observations and investigations prior to chemotherapy is the physical and psychological preparation of the child and his family. The child will, in most circumstances, have a Hickman line catheter inserted in order to avoid the risk of needle phobia (and all its potential long term adverse psychological effects). This provides access for blood sampling, administering cytotoxic therapy and subsequent supportive care, e.g. blood products and intravenous antibiotics. Prior to commencing, time should be spent with the parents and child to explain the treatment. Each should be addressed separately as language appropriate to age may need to be used. The parents often will receive a copy of the protocol. Explanations should include the names of the drugs, their potential complications and a detailed explanation of the problems of bone marrow suppression as the family may be at home when this occurs. Education of the family is a continuous process but the first discussion should be repeated a few days later to ensure comprehension, reiterate important points and allow time for further questions. These interviews are carried out by the consultant or other senior doctor and should be in the presence of a nurse who is often asked further questions or for clarification.

The condition of the child may dictate the timing of the first course of treatment. If his health is deteriorating due to the underlying disease, treatment may be more important than completing the pre-chemotherapy investigations such as CT and bone scans which can wait until later without influencing treatment.

Once all the appropriate investigations have been completed and the family and child are informed about the treatment, the nurse will administer the therapy safely in accordance with predefined guidelines and as the protocol has been prescribed by the medical staff. The nurse must document each drug once administered, including the time and note any immediate adverse effects. Administration of cytotoxic therapy safely is often a time-consuming procedure and this must not be underestimated.

6.5 COMPLICATIONS OF CHEMOTHERAPY

The nursing approach to the commoner complications is summarized in Table 6.1.

Nausea and vomiting

Nausea and vomiting are the most common side effects of patients receiving chemotherapy (Lawrence and Terz, 1977), and in the adult population

Table 6.1 Complications of chemotherapy

Side effect	Nursing intervention	Rationale
1. Anaemia	Observe the patient for: general fatigue, pallor, shortness of breath, headache, dizziness or faintness. Promote rest and position to relieve dyspnoea. Full blood count assessment and transfuse appropriately	To detect early signs of anaemia for prompt treatment
2. Thrombocytopenia	Observe the child for: – petechiae and purpuric areas – fresh ecchymoses – blood in urine, stool, emesis – nose bleeds/gum bleeds Avoid: – rectal thermometers, suppositories – subcutaneous injections – intramuscular injections Full blood count assessment and transfuse appropriately Use of soft toothbrush	Early detection that platelet count may be low requiring transfusion Bleeding may occur due to trauma of the invasive procedure To avoid pain and injury to gums resulting in bleeding when stomatitis is a potential complication
3. Neutropenia	Monitor temperature, pulse, respiration and blood pressure Observe: i. inflammation/redness ii. venous access sites iii. any known/potential foci of infection, e.g. wounds, and swab if necessary	To detect early signs of infection and treat promptly to prevent overwhelming septicaemia (N.B. There will be a lack of pus in the absence of white cells)

Action	Rationale
Avoid: Rectal thermometers	To reduce risk of introducing organisms
Full blood count and administer intravenous antibiotics as prescribed by medical staff	
Pay attention to patient's personal hygiene and educate the family	

Gastrointestinal Tract

1. Anorexia

Action	Rationale
Encourage nutrition sensitively – refer to dietitian – monitor weight	To promote good balanced diet Prevent weight loss Weight gain promotion Tempting child to eat
Meals provided to be small and attractive with high calorie snacks, drinks	
Encourage mouth care Artificial saliva	Promote salivary flow and reduce 'bad tastes'

2. Mouth

Action	Rationale
Examination of mouth – stomatitis – mucositis – inflammation/oedema – plaque – ulcers	To detect any early signs of oral cavity complications in order to prevent or minimise further deterioration
Analgesia/topical anaesthetics Mouthcare Dummy/artificial saliva Nutritional status	Promote pain control for effective mouth care to continue to prevent oral complications initially. If complications occur, mouthcare, artificial saliva etc. – aims to cleanse mouth and keep oral cavity moist and infection free

Table 6.1 *Continued*

Side effect	Nursing intervention	Rationale
3. Stomach		
Nausea	Oral stimulation/mouthcare Antiemetics administration	To promote clean, moist mouth Prevent nausea and vomiting
Vomiting	Nutrition – little and often – bland diet	To provide inviting food in small quantities Large meals will immediately be rejected
	Fluids and electrolyte estimations	Early signs of malnourishment may be detected and electrolyte imbalance can be corrected before dangerous levels are shown biochemically
4. Bowel	Assess 'normal' bowel pattern on admission	Knowledge of abnormal bowel pattern will be determined quickly with this assessment. Prompt treatment can be initiated
		Excess volumes must be reported as fluid balance may become crucial with large volumes of diarrhoea
		Negative balances will be detected promptly and child's chemistry corrected safely before life threatening levels are detected

occurs in up to 83% of patients (Moran *et al.*, 1979). The incidence in the paediatric population is less well documented. However, it is clear that those patients who experience severe nausea and vomiting as a result of their chemotherapy, may experience even more severe nausea and vomiting with subsequent courses (Nesse *et al.*, 1980). It is important, therefore, to control these side effects as early as possible during treatment in order to minimize the potential onset of anticipatory symptoms.

There are few studies of nausea and vomiting associated with chemotherapy specifically in children (Frick *et al.*, 1988) but it is suggested that it is age related. The younger the child, the less likely vomiting is to occur, perhaps due to lack of insight into the treatment-related side effects and of preconceived ideas of how to behave, which the teenager will learn quickly. At any age children rapidly learn behaviour and if the first chemotherapy experience in these terms is negative, it may be difficult to reverse this behaviour. Anticipatory vomiting is particularly hard to control.

Some studies (Headley, 1987) suggest that chemotherapy administered overnight produces less nausea and vomiting than when administered during the day. However, such studies are small and show little difference between the two groups. Large studies need to address this question so that nursing practice can be modified if appropriate. Administration of a wide range of antiemetics, alone or in combination, can be successful in controlling the side effects of chemotherapy (Rhodes *et al.*, 1984). Knowledge of the emetogenicity of individual drugs is important. Some chemotherapy agents appear non-emetogenic in children (e.g. etoposide, vincristine, low dose cytosine). Thus antiemetics can be withheld and treatment can be given in the out-patient department.

Other drugs vary in their degree of emetogenicity. It may be tempting to withhold antiemetics with less emetogenic drugs and give antiemetics only if vomiting occurs. The danger in this is that a cycle of vomiting can occur which is difficult to break. With some chemotherapy regimens, if vomiting can be controlled, treatment may be given on an out-patient basis. For such regimens the child should be admitted for the first course, with intravenous antiemetics given initially, and all subsequent doses given orally as if the child were at home. If this proves successful, subsequent courses will not require admission to hospital. It is clear that antiemetics should be administered prior to chemotherapy rather than just as intervention (Cocket, 1971).

Standard antiemetics (dosage according to weight of the child) include metoclopramide (Maxolon) with dexamethasone (Table 6.2). In adults, high dose metoclopramide, usually as a 24-hour continuous infusion (1–4 mg/kg), has been shown to be the most effective antiemetic with cisplatin (Gralla *et al.*, 1981). This dose is rarely used in children due to the higher incidence of extrapyramidal side effects (Marshall *et al.*, 1989).

Ondansetron, a more recent antiemetic, is very effective in combination with dexamethasone, with minimal side effects (Marty *et al.*, 1990; Pinkerton *et al.*, 1990). Highly emetic cytotoxic drugs, including cisplatin, high dose melphalan and ifosfamide, are now effectively controlled at all ages including the teenagers who are more likely to experience this side effect. Other antiemetics include cyclizine (Valoid), prochlorperazine (Stemetil), domperidone (Motilium) and lorazepam (Ativan). For some patients it will be a case of trial and error in attempting to control vomiting. Procyclidine (Kemadrin) may be given when administering phenothiazines and metoclopramide to prevent dystonic reactions (Table 6.2). One strategy of antiemetics taking into account the degree of emetogenicity is given below:

Regimens of low emetogenicity

Vincristine, vinblastine, chlorambucil, oral cyclophosphamide, oral etoposide, low dose cytarabine.

Antiemetic schedule recommended: None routinely required
If symptoms develop then
metoclopramide $10\,mg/m^2$
p.o. q.d.s.

Table 6.2 Antiemetics (single dosages)

Drug	Route	10–15 kg	15–25 kg	25–40 kg
Metoclopramide	p.o./i.v.	2.5 mg	5 mg	10 mg
Dexamethasone	p.o./i.v.	1 mg	2 mg	4 mg
Chlorpromazine	p.o./i.v.	3.125 mg	6.25 mg	12.5 mg
Lorazepam	p.o./i.v.	0.5 mg	1 mg	2 mg
Prochlorperazine	i.v.	3.125 mg	6.25 mg	12.5 mg
	p.o.	2.5 mg	10 mg	
Ondansetron	i.v.	$4\,mg/m^2$ 12-hourly		
	p.o.	$4\,mg/m^2$ to nearest tablet size 12 hourly		

Note: 1. These doses can be given up to 4-hourly.
   2. Watch for dystonic reactions with metoclopramide and prochlorperazine. If these occur use:
   Procyclidine i.m./i.v. 0.5–2 mg (up to 2 years)
   2–5 mg (2–10 years)
   5–10 mg (over 10 years)
   – single dose, may be repeated after 20 minutes

Regimens of moderate emetogenicity

Combinations containing intravenous cyclophosphamide, doxorubicin, actinomycin D and carboplatin.

Antiemetic schedule recommended
Dexamethasone $4\,mg/m^2$ by slow i.v. injection with chemotherapy then
Dexamethasone $2\,mg/m^2$ t.d.s. p.o. for 2 days
Metoclopramide $10\,mg/m^2$ q.d.s. for 3 days

Oral antiemetic therapy should be prescribed as above to **prevent** delayed emesis, **not** p.r.n.!

Regimens of high emetogenicity

These include cisplatin $\geqslant 50\,mg/m^2$, high dose melphalan and ifosfamide. In this setting ondansetron can produce complete control of emesis in >50% of patients. These results, however, only apply to the control of acute emesis (within 24 hr of chemotherapy). Adding dexamethasone to ondansetron improves the control of acute emesis but dexamethasone and metoclopramide are the most useful agents to treat delayed emesis (Jones *et al.*, 1991).

Recommended schedules

Ondansetron $4\,mg/m^2$ i.v. with each dose of chemotherapy then $4\,mg/m^2$ p.o. (to nearest tablet size), or i.v. if inpatient, 12 hours later.
Dexamethasone $4\,mg/m^2$ orally with chemotherapy then
Dexamethasone $2\,mg/m^2$ p.o. t.d.s. for 2 days ⎫ following completion
Metoclopramide $10\,mg/m^2$ p.o. q.d.s. for 3 days ⎭ of chemotherapy
(See Figure 6.9.)

Antiemetics must be given regularly and continued for some time after cessation of cytotoxic therapy. Their duration will be on an individual basis depending on cytotoxic drugs given and the child himself. At least 24 hours post-emetic cytotoxic drugs is the minimum. Those children who received drugs with known delayed emesis, e.g. cisplatin, or who have a history of delayed emesis following other chemotherapy, should take oral antiemetics home with adequate advice to telephone if vomiting persists despite these measures. Occasionally parents may administer antiemetics such as Maxolon by suppository.

Unfortunately, protracted vomiting can become a great problem despite the above measures. For such children, alternative methods such as scopolamine patches, TENS (transepidermal nerve stimulation) or acupuncture may be useful. For younger children, distraction and relaxation therapies may also have a role (Sauers *et al.*, 1982).

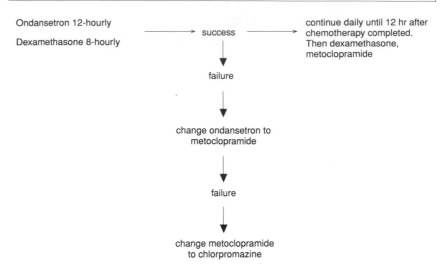

Figure 6.9 Standard regimen for highly emetogenic therapy.

For the child who is vomiting, other nursing care and observations must be considered. Fluid and electrolyte imbalance may occur, thus the child with severe vomiting should be maintained on a fluid balance chart with input and output and weight recorded daily. It may even become necessary to commence intravenous hydration if the child is unable to tolerate diet and fluids, in order to prevent dehydration. Serum electrolytes should be estimated, as potassium loss may be considerable and require replacement. Nutritional deficits may also occur with associated weight loss. A dietitian should be involved and a high calorie, high protein diet encouraged to maintain the child's weight when the child is able to tolerate food. Attention to the mouth is important. After vomiting the child should be encouraged to clean his mouth – not only to clear the mouth of any debris but also promote patient comfort in terms of taste and freshness.

The psychological effect of prolonged vomiting, inability to tolerate diet and weight loss should not be underestimated. These may cause prolonged hospitalization, which compounds feelings of loss of normality. Management of such circumstances requires sensitivity to the situation, listening skills and encouragement and appropriate optimism.

Nausea and vomiting are very distressing side effects of chemotherapy and particularly in the adolescent can be responsible for discontinuation of treatment. They may cause delay in treatments, necessitating extra time for the child to improve nutritional status prior to the next course of treatment.

Diarrhoea

Diarrhoea may be caused by the direct effect of cytotoxic agents on the rapidly dividing epithelial cells of the gastrointestinal tract. Cellular damage causes fluid loss and hypermobility. Diarrhoea usually occurs within a few days of the drug, although in some cases earlier or later.

Nursing care is aimed at monitoring the child's fluid and electrolyte balance, treatment of any imbalance, caring for the child's comfort in terms of pain and cleanliness and assessing and attending to nutritional deficits should they occur.

The volume of diarrhoea will be variable, with some cytotoxic drugs causing more than others, for example, high dose cytarabine, particularly in combination with anthracyclines. The volume of diarrhoea may vary from very little to litres. If possible, separation of urine output from stools should be attempted. The volume, appearance, colour and consistency of the motion must be monitored. Diarrhoea may occur at the nadir of the cycle in the presence of thrombocytopenia, thus blood may be visible. Parents should be warned that this may occur and sloughing of the gastrointestinal lining may be present, which may be very frightening. In these circumstances platelets should be kept above $50 \times 10^9/l$ in an attempt to avoid large bleeds. Fluid balance charts with frequent assessments are essential. Intravenous fluids may be necessary to replace diarrhoeal loss if severe. Clinical signs of dehydration should be regularly sought. Body weight must be recorded at least daily. Electrolyte assessments are made daily, or as often as the child's condition dictates, and imbalances corrected. Albumin and potassium loss may be great in severe cases of chemotherapy-induced diarrhoea. The former may necessitate albumin infusions.

In order to promote patient comfort, antispasmodics for abdominal pain may be administered. Antidiarrhoeals such as loperamide or codeine phosphate to reduce frequency of episodes are also useful. Advice on diet in terms of high calorie food is important as well as omitting high fibre foods, such as bran and fruit, which will worsen the problem. Local hygiene is paramount with gentle cleansing of the perianal region using water and patting dry, in order to prevent excoriation and breakdown of the skin.

If the child or adolescent experiences this distressing side effect, the above nursing intervention must be carried out, but sensitivity for the patient's dignity must be maintained throughout.

Mucositis

Mucositis refers to the inflammation of the mucous membranes due to the effects of chemotherapy on the rapidly dividing cells. Stomatitis refers to this process within the oral cavity, oesophagitis within the oesophagus and mucositis of the intestinal tract is assumed to be occurring at the same time, characterized by proctitis, diarrhoea and abdominal pain.

Up to 40% of patients receiving chemotherapy will develop complications of the oral cavity as a result of cytotoxic therapy (Sonis, Sonis and Liebeman, 1978). It is a particular problem after high doses of anthracyclines, cytarabine and actinomycin D, or if inadequate folinic acid rescue is used after high dose methotrexate. Mucositis is less common after alkylating agents, e.g. cyclophosphamide or cisplatin, but will invariably occur at very high dose, e.g. melphalan (Dreizen, Boday and Rodriques, 1978). Radiotherapy to the head and neck can be expected to exacerbate this problem.

Tissue damage can occur as early as 5–7 days post administration of chemotherapy; the mouth may begin to look pale and dry and erythematous in appearance. The tongue appears coated with raised red papillae. Pain may already be present at this stage, described as a burning sensation. The membranes of cheeks have a corrugated or ridging appearance. The condition of the mouth may progress to having white plaques, severe inflammation and ulceration with associated severe pain. Dysphagia with the sensation of 'having a lump' in the throat when swallowing is often reported (Nunally, Donaghue and Yasko, 1983). The lips also appear dry, cracked and sore and in the presence of thrombocytopenia bleeding often occurs. Xerostomia and taste changes are distressing side effects at this time. The patient may be able to tolerate fluids but not food. However, it is not unusual for the child to be unable to tolerate any diet or fluids and nutritional deficits will ensue if nutritional needs are not considered early.

The child's comfort and nutritional status is without doubt of great importance but, of even more importance is the significance of mucositis in the presence of pancytopenia. Superinfection is a potential fatal complication during this time. As the integrity of the oral cavity is interrupted, opportunistic infection has a portal of entry into the systemic circulation and may cause a life threatening septicaemia. *Klebsiella*, *Escherichia coli*, *Proteus* and *Pseudomonas* species are the most common bacteria of the oral cavity which may cause problems. However, viral infections, especially herpes simplex and fungal infections, such as *Candida albicans* are equally serious in these circumstances.

Mouthcare is an important nursing issue as regards introducing the procedure to the family, ensuring that it is carried out effectively and supporting parents if they choose to be primary care givers for this procedure. However, team work between both medical and nursing staff is essential. Doctors will be prescribers of medications and therefore although the hospitalized child's mouth will be assessed at least daily by the medical staff, the nursing staff will be assessing the condition of the mouth more frequently. The early reporting of new complications is essential.

The aim of mouthcare is to moisten and cleanse the mouth regularly, removing any potential predisposing site for infection (debris) and maintain the integrity of the mucous membranes. Secondly, it is to detect any complication early so that prompt treatment can be instigated. Lastly, in the case of severe oral toxicity, the aim is to treat as prescribed, promote comfort and relief from pain and eventually promote healing until the mouth is healthy, clean and moist again.

It is believed that early intervention with mouthcare probably decreases the incidence of oral complications. During the first few days of admission, the child will be gradually settling into the hospital routine and beginning to trust the staff taking care of him. Ideally, his 'special nurse' will build up enough trust to teach him and his family the cleansing of the mouth. Mouthcare should not be a painful experience in the healthy mouth and compliance, with time, is easily possible. Demonstrating the procedure on 'dolly', 'mummy' or his nurse as well as seeing all the other children routinely cleaning their mouths are all positive reinforcements. It is extremely important for the child to be accustomed to the procedure whilst he is well and not in pain, so that if mucositis does occur the procedure will continue as a routine and not another alien intervention whilst he is already feeling unwell.

Mouth assessment should begin from the day of the child's admission (a child with leukaemia, already pancytopenic, may present with mucositis and ulceration). Compliance, particularly in the very young takes time and experience shows that most children will open their mouth for assessment as soon as trust is gained. The use of a torch is essential. Children do not respond well to spatula in the mouth, thus a gloved finger to gently view inside the cheeks is more effective. Some children prefer to do this themselves. Children are usually able to tell you if they have a problem, so questioning them is important.

There is very little published research into mouthcare. Most literature on the subject suggests that nursing measures to promote a normal, healthy, moist mouth are based on experience. Although nurses may need to refer to local policy for their mouthcare procedure, the practice discussed below has been found to be effective and tolerable.

The tools used for cleaning the mouth are an issue in the pancytopenic patient. A toothbrush remains the instrument of choice for effectively removing debris and plaque. However, it is argued that the abrasiveness of the toothbrush in the neutropenic/thrombocytopenic patient with mucositis could result in injury to the membranes and provide a focus for endogenous infection. Some suggest discontinuation of toothbrush when the neutrophil count falls below $1.0 \times 10^9/l$ and platelets fall below $50 \times 10^9/l$. In the case of the child, he may not tolerate a toothbrush at this stage. However, it may be possible to use a soft toothbrush to remove debris if used extremely cautiously. Foam sticks (toothettes) are used in conjunction to clean palate and gums. Foam sticks are known to be ineffective in removing debris (Hathorn and Pizzo, 1989). The swabbing of the gums, palate and tongue will stimulate salivary flow and cleaning these areas is convenient, hygienic and disposable without causing pain and trauma.

A variety of commercial products exists for the cleansing of the mouth. When these have been examined for effectiveness, it was concluded that frequency and consistency of cleansing is a more important factor than the product used and therefore individual taste and preference should be considered. Of major importance in paediatrics is the toleration of the procedure, as many commercial products are rejected by children on account of their taste and pain to sore areas. Poland (1987) have reported that mouthcare which includes lemon glycerine or alcohol actually dehydrates the mucosa and promotes the growth of bacteria and should be avoided. If the child is old enough to co-operate, he should rinse the mouth without swallowing. This will help remove any debris which may have been dislodged during the procedure.

Antifungal agents such as nystatin and amphotericin B rinses have been shown to be successful in prophylaxis against oral *Candida* (Shepherd, 1978). Children are encouraged to swish and swallow and refrain from drinking for 15–20 minutes.

The lips need to be treated in order to prevent dryness, cracking and pain. The most effective product appears to be yellow soft paraffin/ petroleum jelly which forms an occlusive film and prevents evaporation of moisture. This procedure should be carried out at least four times a day, after meals and prior to bedtime. Suggestions have been made to increase this to 2-hourly during the day. Whilst this should not be discouraged, the sick child with a sore mouth will require numerous other interventions and the child will soon become irritable and non-compliant due to continuous interruptions. Then mouthcare will not be carried out effectively.

The unfortunate 40% who develop mouth complications will often require more aggressive intervention. If the child is febrile, intravenous antibiotics according to local policy will be administered to treat potential bacterial infections. If the white plaques are suspicious of *Candida*, fluconazole may be given but with persistent fever of 72 hours intravenous amphotericin will be prescribed. Ulceration even remotely suspicious of a viral infection, particularly herpes simplex, will be treated with intravenous acyclovir. More recently, sucralfate, which is a palatable elixir, appears to be effective in the healing and relief of pain of ulcers (non-herpetic) by combining with the exudate from the ulcer and promoting healing.

Pain in the child with mucositis is usually made tolerable with paracetamol (Calpol elixir), but when severe requires very strong analgesia. Although many commercial local anaesthetic products exist, such as xylocaine and Difflam, they often cause pain initially before the relief of pain. The young child finds this intolerable, but the older child and teenager sometimes finds this effective. There should be a low threshold to introduce a low dose continuous infusion of diamorphine which provides effective pain control, comfort and allows the child to carry out mouthcare without being too sedated.

The child who requires pain control will often have a dry mouth with altered taste. These children's nutritional deficits must be considered and met (see section on nutrition, Chapter 10). The dietitian will be involved and commonly the child will require total parenteral nutrition during this time.

Parents most commonly assume the role of primary care giver as regards the health of their child's mouth. By working closely with the nursing staff, the parents become expert at carrying out this procedure and learn when to report any deterioration in the condition of their child's mouth. The child will often clean his mouth himself under supervision, and will often clean more thoroughly than the third party, who is worried about causing pain and therefore does not exert so much pressure during cleansing.

It should be remembered, however, that it is primarily the nurse's responsibility and the parents must feel able to opt out. This does not happen often, but during particularly stressful times, when their child's mouth is sore, they may wish for the nurse to do the care for fear of causing pain. They are then available to cuddle their child afterwards.

Mouthcare continues to be a challenge to the oncology nurse. Its importance cannot be over-emphasized, both in terms of patient comfort and in the prevention of potentially fatal septicaemia.

Bone marrow suppression

Bone marrow suppression (myelosuppression) may be a result of the disease process itself, for example, with leukaemia or metastatic disease in the bone marrow, or as a result of treatment. Long term survival in childhood cancer is to a large extent due to very intensive treatment programmes, particularly for previously poor prognosis tumours. The result of these intensive therapies (chemotherapy ± radiotherapy) is a significantly increased risk of the children experiencing severe bone marrow suppression and often for a prolonged period of time. The specialist in paediatric oncology must have a full understanding of the implications of this in order to be able to care for their patient safely and effectively and be able to educate the child's family of this potentially life-threatening complication of the child's treatment.

Neutropenia (Granulocytopenia)

Neutropenia is defined as a reduction in the number of neutrophils (granulocytes) as a percentage of the total white count. White blood cells are responsible for containing and neutralizing invading micro-organisms by migrating to the site of infection (Brown and Kiss, 1983). As the number of neutrophils falls, the incidence of infection increases. However, not only may the number of neutrophils be reduced to a level where infections may be severe, but the function of these cells may be impaired. Patients are at severe risk of infection when the absolute neutrophil count is less than $0.5 \times 10^9/l$ and particularly $<0.2 \times 10^9/l$ (Fox, 1981). Infection is a serious complication and it is the most common cause of death during treatment (Brandt, 1990), thus the importance of prevention, treatment and education cannot be over-emphasized.

Recognition of infection in the neutropenic patient can be very difficult due to the absence of the classic inflammatory response. Localized infection may produce pain and erythema but inflammation and the formation of 'pus' will be absent, and thus the insidious onset of infection requires very close observation.

The myelosuppressed child is very susceptible to both endogenous and exogenous infections. Endogenous microbial flora, for example *Pseudomonas aeruginosa*, *Escherichia coli*, *Klebsiella pneumoniae* and *Candida albicans* may be responsible for as high as 80% of infections in the myelosuppressed patient (Henschel, 1985; Hathorn and Pizzo, 1989). This is to some extent a result of the normal acid and enzyme producing cells which maintain the integrity of the gastrointestinal tract being damaged by chemotherapy and the 'normal flora' is replaced by pathogenic organisms (Adams, 1985; Carlson, 1985; Hathorn and Pizzo, 1989) (Chapter 10).

Nursing management

Management of the neutropenic child includes prevention where possible, and early detection of infection with prompt action and aggressive treatment.

Prevention of infection is often not possible but measures to ensure early diagnosis and treatment begin with education of the whole family. The educator must be a specialist in paediatric oncology and will often be the nurse who has built up a rapport with the child and his family and should be able to assess their degree of comprehension. This may be important in terms of how often the child needs assessing in out-patients, or how often the community nurse needs to do a home visit. Firstly to ensure the child is in good health, and secondly to be able to reiterate important preventative measures already discussed at the hospital.

Exogenous infection may be prevented by minimizing exposure to environmental sources of infection. This means avoiding others with known infections, such as coughs, sore throats and especially chicken pox, shingles and measles. The child should, however, be encouraged to attend school to continue his education, socialization and achieve a sense of normality. Education of the appropriate individuals at school should be completed by the time the child returns and parents well informed of the importance of reporting their child's illness immediately to the school in order that appropriate actions be taken if needed. Crowded areas such as cinemas and shopping centres should be avoided until otherwise advised.

Endogenous infection is difficult to prevent, as it is usually the chemotherapy which affects the integrity of the gastrointestinal tract, giving rise to such infections. However, there are some measures which can be taken in an attempt to minimize the risks.

Maintaining the integrity of the gastrointestinal tract begins with oral hygiene. Consistent cleaning of the mouth at frequent intervals is of paramount importance (see section on mouthcare). It may also be important in detecting early signs of infection if the integrity is broken and ulceration and white patches appear. The condition of the oral cavity is probably indicative of the condition of the rest of the gastrointestinal tract.

Rectal temperature measurement must be avoided in the neutropenic child. Trauma to the rectum by thermometer, suppositories or enemas may result in a tear, loss of integrity and entrance of the gut flora systemically, causing sepsis which may prove life threatening. The perirectal region should be kept scrupulously clean and dry, particularly after bowel motions.

Maintaining the integrity of the skin is equally important. Hygiene advice includes daily baths or, preferably showers, using mild soaps and moisturizing the skin, particularly if dry, in order to prevent cracking, and thus a focus for skin flora to develop into endogenous infection.

Many children receiving intensive chemotherapeutic regimens will have an existing indwelling central line/Hickman catheter. As the exit site is a potential source of infection, aseptic technique should be implemented when dealing with the site according to local policy and any abnormality reported immediately. This also applies to any breaks in the skin which may have occurred from the child having a fall or from invasive procedures, such as lumbar punctures and bone marrow biopsies. The latter are a particular potential problem when performed in the pancytopenic child at diagnosis.

The most important means to attempt to prevent the transmission of exogenous infection is thorough hand washing. This should be emphasized to parents, particularly when dealing with Hickman catheters and dressing of the exit site.

Early detection of infection in these children is essential to prevent life-threatening septicaemia (Brown and Kiss, 1983). Fever is the best single measure of an infection and parents should be informed that under no circumstances should a fever be ignored and contact with the hospital should be made immediately. However, parents should also be advised that if at any time they are unhappy with their child, even if they cannot specifically describe what the problem is, then this is also a good indication for contacting the hospital. Other reasons for the parents to contact the hospital are flushed appearance, rigors, redness/erythema at Hickman exit site or any other wound on their child's body, dysuria, diarrhoea, persistent cough or a sore mouth, with or without white patches or ulcers.

On admission to hospital the child will be assessed, have a full blood count estimated and observations taken. A full infection screen should be carried out which will include blood cultures, urine and stool specimen, swabs from any potential foci of infection which may include venous access swab, throat swab, swab of lesions where a child may have fallen. A chest X-ray should be taken also.

Broad-spectrum antibiotics must be commenced immediately, as awaiting for culture results may result in rapid deterioration in the child. Some patients fail to respond to first-line antibiotics; these are changed according to culture results or electively at 48–72 hours unless the child becomes septically shocked, in which case a change of antibiotics is made at this time. For fevers which have not settled within 4–5 days, opportunistic infections, especially fungal, must be considered and amphotericin B or fluconazole considered (Chapter 10). The duration of antibiotics is according to local policy. Whether the child is culture negative or culture positive will influence the decision. However, in the child who is culture negative some physicians wait until the neutropenia resolves, whilst others require a given number of days that the child is afebrile, arguing that a lengthy course may cause increased risk of drug toxicity and fungal infections due to prolonged suppression of normal gut flora.

The importance of detecting infection in the neutropenic child is paramount and the development of a temperature is an emergency. Sepsis may progress extremely rapidly if not detected and treated early.

Thrombocytopenia

Chemotherapy may suppress the platelet production. It does not affect mature circulating platelets but the stem cells from which they develop. The life span of a platelet is approximately 2–5 days and the platelet count nadir can be expected to occur 10–14 days after chemotherapy, reflecting the maturation time. With some drugs the nadir occurs later, e.g. busulphan or BCNU.

Thrombocytopenia may be defined as a platelet count of less than $100 \times 10^9/l$ (normal platelet count $150–300 \times 10^9/l$). However, in the absence of other factors such as fever or coagulopathy bleeding is rare until the platelet count falls much lower. At $\sim$20 $\times$ 10^9/l the risk increases and if allowed to fall below 5–10 $\times$ 10^9/l, there is a significant risk of bleeding, particularly in the central nervous system and gastrointestinal tract.

Platelets migrate to sites of injury within blood vessels and creating a clot to prevent further blood loss (Wroblewski and Wroblewski, 1981). For the child who has impaired coagulation, nursing management is aimed at prevention of injury, early detection of bleeding and prompt action where required.

Nursing management
The child is often at home at the nadir of the platelet count and parental education is therefore an important nursing task prior to discharge. Parents are advised of the signs of low platelets, such as bruising without a specific injury, petechiae, nose bleeds and bleeding gums. Gastrointestinal bleeding or haematuria in the young will be easy to detect, but the older child and teenager needs to be strongly advised to confide in their parents if this occurs. Avoiding bumping and bruising within the normal daily activities of life is advised and vigorous sports such as rugby and hockey should be avoided. Girls who are menstruating and receiving very myelosuppressive regimens will be given medication such as daily oestrogens to stop this until their treatment has been completed.

Advice on other drugs is very important, particularly as aspirin is a common household medication which must be avoided. Parents are advised to telephone the hospital if they wish to give a medication and are unsure of its safety.

If thrombocytopenia requiring possible platelet transfusion is suspected, a full blood count assessment will be taken. If this is carried out using venepuncture, prolonged pressure will need to be applied to the site in order to avoid a painful haematoma.

Nursing intervention aimed at prevention of trauma which could contribute to a bleed includes: avoidance of rectal thermometers or oral medication which may traumatize mucosa already damaged as a result of chemotherapy; invasive procedures should be avoided if possible during this time including urinary catheterization; soft toothbrushes may need to be temporarily discontinued and toothettes/foam sticks only used if gums are extremely sensitive; injections, subcutaneous or intramuscular, should also be avoided. Awareness of potential sites of bleeding is essential with testing faeces and urine for occult blood if blood is not obviously present. Also observe any sites of invasive procedures, such as Hickman exit site, lumbar puncture and bone marrow site and regularly examine skin, oral mucosa and, with severe thrombocytopenia, the optic fundi.

Platelet transfusions will need to be given to some children. The level at which transfusions are given is generally 20 $\times$ 10^9/l when the risk of bleeding spontaneously increases. However, some centres advocate a lower level ($10-15 \times 10^9$/l) and the child's general condition must obviously be considered. Even with a platelet count of greater than 20×10^9/l some children will be symptomatic and require treatment. It is also important to remember that high temperatures and rigors reduce platelet survival, thus a considerable drop may occur within a 24-hour period. Although bleeding in children receiving chemotherapy is usually due to thrombocytopenia, other clotting factors may be affected and an assessment of the child's coagulation picture should be considered, as other clotting factors such as vitamin K or fresh frozen plasma may stop bleeding (Chapter 10).

The administration of platelet transfusion is not without problems, the most common complication being a temperature associated with a rigor. Premedication of hydrocortisone and chlorpheniramine is successful in preventing this reaction for many (Brager and Yasko, 1984) although platelet filters may need to be used. The latter remove neutrophils from the platelet transfusion which are usually the cause of the reaction. In some cases single donor or HLA matched platelets are required.

Anaemia

The life span of a red blood cell is 120 days, and anaemia, defined as a reduction in the number of circulating red blood cells, is common in the myelosuppressed child. It is rarely an acute problem except following a bleed. Many children will remain asymptomatic with a relatively low haemoglobin level but, in general, if the haemoglobin level falls below 9 g a blood transfusion will be considered. However, if the child has evidence of active bleeding, a transfusion may be required at a higher haemoglobin level. Those children who are symptomatic may look pale and experience fatigue, lethargy and shortness of breath in more severe anaemia. Nursing management is directed towards educating parents into recognizing these symptoms at home and control of symptoms in the hospital. Pending transfusion the anaemic child will require promotion of rest which may be achieved by providing interesting activities which can be done whilst the child physically rests, e.g. arts and crafts, computer games.

Symptoms are reversed after transfusion of blood and the child is cared for during the blood transfusion as for the administration of any blood products. The nurse must be aware of the potential complications and all the necessary resuscitation measures readily available.

Other complications

Acute toxicity to various organs is summarized in Table 6.3. Late effects of chemotherapy are reviewed in Chapter 12.

Table 6.3 Organ toxicity

	Marrow	Mucositis	Intestine	Liver	Kidney	Heart	Neurological	Lung	Gonad	Alopecia
Methotrexate	+	+	+	+	+*	−	+	+*	−	−
5FU	+	−	−	−	−	−	−	−	−	−
Cytarabine	+	+	+	+	−	−	+*	−	−	−
6TG	+	−	−	+	−	−	−	−	−	−
Cyclophosphamide	+	−	−	−	−	+*	−	−	+	+
Ifosfamide	+	−	−	−	+	+†	+	−	+	+
CCNU	+	−	−	−	−	−	−	−	+	−
Cisplatin	−	−	−	+*	+	−	+*	+	−	+
Vincristine	−	−	+	−	−	−	+	−	−	−
Vinblastine	+	−	−	−	−	−	+	−	−	−
Etoposide	+	+	−	−	−	−	−	−	−	+
Doxorubicin	+	+	+	+	−	+	−	−	−	+
Daunorubicin	+	+	+	+	−	+	−	−	−	+
Actinomycin	+	+	+	−	−	−	−	−	−	+
Bleomycin	−	−	−	−	−	−	−	+	−	−
DTIC	+	+	−	−	−	−	−	−	−	−
Procarbazine	+	−	−	−	−	−	−	−	+	−
Amsacrine	+	+	+	−	−	−	−	−	−	+
Chlorambucil	+	−	−	−	−	−	−	−	+	−
Asparaginase	−	−	−	+/−	−	−	+/−	−	−	−

* at high dose
† may exacerbate doxorubicin cardiotoxicity

REFERENCES

Adams, A. (1985) External barrier to infection. *Nursing Clinics of North America*, **20**(1), 145–149.

Ames, B.M., McCann, J. and Yamaski, E. (1975) Carcinogens are mutagens: A simple test system. *Mutational Research*, **33**, 27–28.

Brager, B.L. and Yasko, J.M. (1984) *Care of the Client Receiving Chemotherapy* (ed. V. Reston) Reston Publishing Co., Virginia, pp. 96–180.

Brandt, B. (1990) Nursing protocol for the patient with neutropenia. *Oncology Nursing Forum*, **17**(1), 9–14.

Brown, M.H. and Kiss, M.E. (1983) Quality assurance. Standards of clinical nursing practice for leukaemia, neutropenia and thrombocytopenia. *Cancer Nursing*, **6**, 487–494.

Carlson, A.C. (1985) Infection prophylaxis in the patient with cancer. *Oncology Nursing Forum*, **12**(3), 56–63.

Cocket, R. (1971) Antiemetics. *Practitioner*, **206**, 56–63.

Dreizen, S., Boday, C. and Rodriques, V. (1978) Oral complications of cancer chemotherapy. *Postgraduate Medicine*, **58**, 76.

Fox, L.S. (1981) Granulocytopenia in the adult cancer patients. *Cancer Nursing*, **6**, 487–494.

Frick, S.A., Delpo, E.G., Keith, J.A., Davis, M.S. (1988) Chemotherapy associated nausea and vomiting in paediatric oncology patients. *Cancer Nursing*, **11**(2), 118–124.

Gralla, R.J., Itri, L.M., Pisko, S.E. *et al.* (1981) Antiemetic efficacy of high-dose metoclopramide: Randomized trials with placebo and prochlorperazine in patients with chemotherapy-induced nausea and vomiting. *New England Journal of Medicine*, **305**, 905–909.

Hathorn, J. and Pizzo, P. (1989) Infectious complications in the paediatric cancer patient, in *Paediatric Oncology* (eds P.A. Pizzo and D.G. Poplack) Lippincott, Philadelphia, pp. 837–867.

Headley, J. (1987) The influence of administration time on chemotherapy induced nausea and vomiting. *Oncology Nursing Forum*, **14**(16), 43–47.

Henschel, L. (1985) Fever patterns in the neutropenic patient. *Cancer Nursing*, **8**(6), 301–305.

Jones, A.L., Hill, A.S., Soukop, M. *et al.* (1991) Comparison of dexamethasone and ondansetron in the prophylaxis of emesis induced by moderately emetogenic chemotherapy. *Lancet*, **338**, 483–487.

Lawrence, J. and Terz, J.J. (1977) *Cancer Management.* Grune and Stratton, New York.

Marshall, G., Kerr, S., Vowels, M. *et al.* (1989) Antiemetic therapy for chemotherapy-induced vomiting: Metoclopramide, benztropine, dexamethasone, and lorazepam regimen compared with chlorpromazine alone. *Journal of Pediatrics*, **115**, 156–160.

Marty, M., Pouillart, P., Scholl, S. *et al.* (1990) Comparison of the 5-hydroxy-tryptamine$_3$ (serotonin) antagonist ondansetron (GR 38032F) with high-dose metoclopramide in the control of cisplatin-induced emesis. *New England Journal of Medicine*, **322**, 816–821.

Moran, C., Smith, D.C., Anderson, D.A., McArdle, C.S. (1979) Incidence of nausea and vomiting with cytotoxic chemotherapy. A prospective randomised trial of antiemetics. *British Medical Journal*, **15**, 1322–1324.

Nesse, R.M., Carli, T., Curtis, G.C. and Kleinman, P.D. (1980) Pretreatment nausea in cancer chemotherapy. A conditioned response? *Psychosomatic Medicine*, **17**, 33–36.

Nunally, C., Donaghue, M. and Yasko, J.M. (1983) Esophagitis in *Guidelines for cancer care: symptom management* (ed. J.M. Yasko) Reston Publishing Co., Virginia, USA.

Pinkerton, C.R., Williams, D., Wootton, C. *et al.* (1990) 5-HT$_3$ antagonist ondansetron – an effective outpatient antiemetic in cancer treatment. *Archives of Disease in Childhood*, **65**, 822–825.

Poland, J.M. (1987) Comparing More-stir to lemon swabs. *American Journal of Nursing*, **87**, 87.

Rhodes, V.A., Watson, P.M. and Johnson, M.H. (1984) Development of reliable and valid measure of nausea and vomiting. *Cancer Nursing*, **7**(1), 33–41.

Sauers, S. *et al.* (1982) The challenge of physical care, in *Nursing Care of the Child with Cancer* (eds D. Fochtman and G. Toley), Little, Brown & Co., Boston.

Shepherd, J.P. (1978) The management of the oral complications of leukaemia. *Oral Surgery*, **45**, 543–548.

Sonis, S.T., Sonis, A.L. and Liebeman, A. (1978) Oral complications in patients receiving treatment for malignancies other than of the head and neck. *Journal of the American Dental Association*, **97**, 464–471.

Wroblewski, S.S. and Wroblewski, S.H. (1981) Caring for the patient with chemotherapy-induced thrombocytopenia. *American Journal of Nursing*, **81**(4), 746.

7 | Radiotherapy

Radiotherapy has been used as a form of cancer treatment for almost a century. It is rarely the sole treatment in paediatrics as most children's tumours have potential for metastases and therefore radiotherapy alone will not be curative. It is, however, common in combination with chemotherapy and/or surgery. It may also be used primarily to treat oncological emergencies, for example spinal cord compression.

Radiotherapy is the delivery of ionizing radiation to cause cell damage or destruction. Ionization is the destabilization of the electrical neutrality of the atom. The nucleus of an atom contains protons (positive electrical charge), electrons (negative electrical charge) and neutrons (no electrical charge). It is the removal of orbiting electrons by a beam of radiation that causes the destabilization of the atom.

The biological consequence of these atomic alterations is to cause damage to DNA. This includes single-strand breaks, double-strand breaks and damage to the pyrimidine bases. This damage may be severe enough to prevent cell division or cause cell death. There is also an indirect damaging effect due to the ionization of cellular water. This causes the release of toxic 'free radicals' such as atomic oxygen $[O^-]$.

The main types of radiation used in paediatrics are:

1. X-rays – delivered by linear accelerator, and gamma rays – emitted from a radioactive isotope in the form of a sealed or unsealed source, for example cobalt. The radiation in X-ray and gamma radiation (photons) differs only in the way they are produced: X-rays indirectly and gamma rays directly. Linear accelerators produce radiation by firing electrons from an electron gun into an accelerator tube. An electrical field sweeps the electrons along the tube which are then directed onto a target, for example tungsten, and emitted as X-rays.
2. Beta particles – emitted from radioactive isotopes and used in sealed or unsealed forms. An isotope is an atom where the number of neutrons differs from the number of electrons and protons. This im-

balance causes instability in the nucleus and as the nucleus tries to restabilize it may break up or decay, thus producing radioactivity. Such radio-isotopes either occur naturally, for example iridium and plutonium, or can be produced by bombarding isotopes with neutrons in a nuclear reactor, for example cobalt, iodine, caesium, gold, iridium.
3. Electron beam – produced directly by a linear accelerator.

The radiation emitted from a radio-isotope lessens with time. The term 'half-life' is used to describe the amount of time taken for the rate of radioactivity emitted to fall to half. An example is ^{131}iodine, the half-life of which is eight days. Units in radiotherapy relate either to the amount of energy imparted in relation to mass or the number of disintegrations occurring in an isotope. One gray (Gy) is equivalent to 1 joule/kg but centigray (cGy) are usually used, e.g. the dose for a sarcoma will be around 40–50 cGy. One Curie (Ci) = 3.7×10^{10} disintegrations/second (the decay of 1 g of radium).

Radiotherapy may be administered externally (teletherapy) in which a beam of radiation is delivered from a distance, or internally (brachytherapy) in which the radiation is administered close to the tumour in the form of sealed source. A third technique uses systemically delivered radio-isotope which is taken up by the tumour target. The type of radiation used and the method of delivery will depend on the tumour type and site. Orthovoltage or supervoltage (beam energy <1 meV) is rarely used due to the high dose received by the skin. With megavoltage machines – either gamma radiation from a cobalt source or photons from a linear accelerator – the maximum dose is delivered at a deeper tissue level. For superficial tumours electron beam therapy can be delivered much closer to the surface. Alternatively, brachytherapy may be appropriate with delivery of either photons or particulate irradiation (Figure 7.1).

7.1 THE EFFECTS OF TREATMENT

Within the treatment field radiotherapy causes damage to normal cells as well as malignant cells. It causes greatest damage to dividing cells and therefore tissues with a fast proliferation rate, such as bone marrow, gastrointestinal tract, epithelium, skin and hair follicles are particularly sensitive to radiation. These show acute reactions but are generally able to repair quickly and the damage is therefore not usually permanent. Tissue that does not proliferate or with a slow proliferation rate, such as the brain, spinal cord and kidney may show late reactions which may be irreversible.

The side effects and degree of damage are dependent on several factors

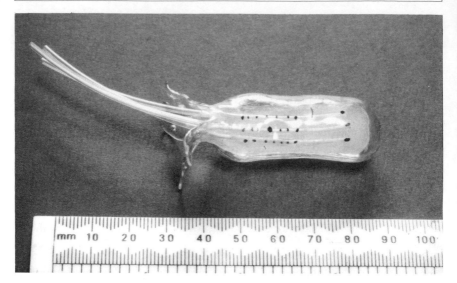

Figure 7.1 Mould containing iridium radioactive source. This was made specifically for a young girl with a small amount of residual rhabdomyosarcoma in the vaginal wall.

including the type of radiation, its dose, the duration and frequency of treatment, the volume and anatomical site treated and finally the individual patient's maturation tolerance level. Organs that are irradiated during their maturation are more susceptible to radiation damage than those that have completed their development. The age of the child is also an important factor. Growth retardation and asymmetry can be expected if bone or soft tissue are irradiated during early life.

The use of combined modality treatment has facilitated lower radiation doses. Chemotherapy has proved to be very effective in the treatment of paediatric tumours, such as Wilms', rhabdomyosarcoma and Hodgkin's disease and has resulted in the need for lower radiation doses and smaller treatment volumes. Randomized studies have demonstrated that with many chemosensitive tumours it can be omitted altogether.

Tumours of the central nervous system is one tumour group, however, where chemotherapy has not had the same results and radiotherapy is still the main treatment modality. The central nervous system experiences a time of rapid growth and development (myelination) during the first 2–3 years of life but by the age of 5 years maturation is almost complete. Irradiation of the central nervous system before myelination is complete can produce irreversible damage affecting intellectual and endocrine function (Kun *et al.*, 1990).

Side effects from radiotherapy can be acute and occur at the time of radiation or develop later. The early side effects include bone marrow depression, alopecia, nausea and vomiting and skin reactions, but are dependent upon the area being irradiated. The late side effects that children are at risk of developing include abnormal growth and development of tissue, abnormal function of organs and the induction of second malignancies (Tait, 1992).

7.2 PREPARATION FOR TREATMENT

Generally children receive radiotherapy in the form of teletherapy. Children with neuroblastoma may receive treatment using an unsealed radio-isotope, ^{131}I meta-iodobenzylguanidine (mIBG) and with rhabdomyosarcomas radiation treatment is occasionally given in the form of a sealed radio-isotope such as caesium or iridium. The preparation, care and side effects differ to those from teletherapy and will be discussed later.

Adults have many misconceptions about radiotherapy. They are aware of its carcinogenic effect and often display negative attitudes to its use (Peck and Boland, 1977). As previously mentioned, children are sensitive to the anxieties of their parents so it is important to discuss any fears or anxieties that the parents may have about the treatment and reassure them by sharing information with them. The type of information required includes the goal of treatment, the type of treatment, the length of time involved, both for the administration of individual fractions and the number of fractions, for example how many days or weeks. The likely side effects and any potential problems should also be discussed. Parents and patients need to be aware that occasionally the effects of the radio therapy may mimic the presenting signs or symptoms of the disease and thus avoid unnecessary worry that the disease is progressing.

Radiotherapy is one form of treatment that the patients must receive alone. Patients receiving external beam radiation must be able to lie still in a specific position alone in a room dominated by a large piece of equipment. The use of intercoms and two-way television circuits have made tremendous impact in enabling patients to cope, but for many young children being able to hear or see their significant carer on a TV screen is not sufficient.

Facilitating children to cope with this form of treatment requires a flexible approach. Assessment of the child's ability will be to some extent dependent upon his age and his level of development, but will also include the position he must adopt for the treatment, the length of time it takes, any previous experiences including having watched fellow patients receiving their treatment and his general physical and emotional well being.

The participation of the play therapist during the assessment and preparation of the patient is vital. Visits to the department, meeting key people, observing the machinery, practising with the intercom and television, observing another child receiving their treatment may be useful to some patients. Information booklets and photograph albums are also very useful. The treatment of children who after assessment are thought to be unable to comply with the restrictions may be carried out under sedation or using a general anaesthesia such as ketamine.

The main advantage of the short-acting anaesthesia is to ensure that the children are able to resume their normal daily activities more quickly than if sedation is used. Central venous devices may be placed to facilitate the administration of daily i.v. anaesthesia and avoid daily intramuscular injections.

Children receiving cranial irradiation require a perspex helmet to ensure accurate alinement and positioning. The making of the helmet or mould can be frightening and distressing for children and parents. Before a perspex mould is produced a plaster cast mould of the child's head has to be made. Some children find this more distressing than the treatment and again sedation or anaesthesia may be required. Parents and personnel can be with the child during this procedure and may, therefore, enable the child to cope. Again, the playtherapist is vital in the preparation for this procedure. Plastercast moulds on dolls provide the child with the opportunity to act out fears or anxieties that he or she may have.

Before the treatment can be implemented it must first be planned and simulated. The simulator reproduces radiotherapy treatment by using X-rays instead of high energy beams. The angles of the radiation beams and the beam size are planned and CT or MRI images taken to show the tumour volume. The location of the appropriate lead shields to prevent the patient being exposed to unnecessary radiation is planned. The planning procedure takes much longer than the individual treatments and again children may require sedation or anaesthesia to cope. Planning and further simulation may be required as treatment progresses.

Most children will receive radiotherapy as outpatients. Even those requiring daily anaesthesia or sedation may be treated as day cases. Determining a specific time for the treatment enables the family to set some form of routine. Children requiring daily anaesthetics benefit from receiving treatment early in the morning, i.e. 9.00 a.m., as they may not tolerate fasting for long and can have a delayed breakfast once the treatment is completed. Sedation is better carried out at the end of the day so that the child does not sleep through normal daily activities. A multidisciplinary team approach is vital in planning the care for the whole family. Some children are able to continue attending school during their course of treatment, others may need support from the ward school teacher or require home tuition. Financial support may be needed to meet the cost of additional travelling expenses, time off work or help with the rest of the family.

7.3 ACUTE SIDE EFFECTS

As previously mentioned the main side effects that occur reflect the area being irradiated. However, many patients do experience some general side effects including fatigue and malaise, anorexia, nausea and vomiting. The cause of these symptoms may be related to metabolic effects of tumour breakdown, bone marrow depression and the reaction to anxiety and stress. Preparation and education about the side effects is vital to enable the child and his family to set realistic goals and to plan their participation during the treatment.

Scalp

Alopecia will occur only in the area of the treatment field. The degree of hair loss is dependent upon the dose of radiation. Less than 30 Gy will cause thinning or partial hair loss only. It will regrow once the treatment is completed. However, at greater than 45 Gy the hair loss will be complete and the loss may be permanent. If the hair loss is partial, patients may require advice on techniques to conceal the area using restyling methods, wigs or hair pieces. Advice on scalp care is necessary. The use of a head covering is important to avoid sunburn, as this can aggravate the side effects of the radiation on the scalp. Excessive hair brushing and the use of tight hair bands should be avoided to prevent further irritations to the scalp (general skin care will be discussed later).

Brain

As previously mentioned, the commencement of radiotherapy can cause an increase in symptoms due to oedema. Thus children receiving cranial irradiation for a brain tumour may develop signs of raised intracranial pressure due to cerebral oedema. This is usually for a short period of time only but may require dexamethasone or occasionally mannitol.

Other acute side effects of cranial irradiation include headache, nausea and vomiting. A 'somnolence syndrome' with fatigue, occasionally signs of meningism, and often a low-grade fever occur 6–8 weeks after cranial irradiation. Its mechanism is unclear but it may be eased with oral steroids, although this is rarely required.

Mouth

If the oral cavity and salivary gland fall within the treatment fields the patient and family will require specific education and advice about mouth care and nutrition.

Radiation parotitis (swollen, painful salivary glands) can occur after 1 or 2 fractions of radiotherapy. A mild analgesic such as paracetamol is usually sufficient to control symptoms. The saliva may become more viscous and reduced in quantity. Patients are advised to increase their oral fluid intake and avoid dry foods (nutrition is covered in detail in Chapter 10). However, it is important to remember that saliva contains natural defences against tooth decay and therefore an alteration or reduction in saliva will increase the risk of dental problems and calls for oral hygiene programmes that the patient is likely to comply with.

Oral cavity

Erythema of the oral mucosa may occur after 2 Gy. Regeneration of epithelial cells occurs 7–14 days after the completion of irradiation. Mouth care programmes must, therefore, be carried out after the cessation of treatment.

Gastrointestinal tract

Dysphagia may occur as a complication of radiation to the mediastinum, for example with Hodgkin's lymphoma. Dietary advice and the use of analgesic and gargles are useful. Nausea and vomiting may occur if the stomach is in the field of treatment. Regular anti-emetics prior to and post radiotherapy are advisable as are alternative methods, for example diversional therapy, deep breathing exercises and relaxation. Again, dietary advice is extremely valuable and should include the type and timing of meals, avoidance of sight and smells that aggravate the symptoms and regular assessment of the patient's nutritional, fluid and electrolyte state.

Irradiation of the bowel, for example in Wilms' tumour or neuroblastoma may cause signs and symptoms of nausea and vomiting, diarrhoea and cramping (small intestine) and frequent diarrhoea with pain (large intestine). These symptoms may persist for 7–14 days following the completion of treatment. Antidiarrhoeal agents and/or analgesics such as codeine or opiates, which also help to reduce diarrhoea, are recommended. Appropriate nutritional advice must also be given and the patient's nutritional, electrolyte and fluid status must again be regularly assessed.

Pelvis

Acute cystitis, for example associated with treatment of a large pelvic Ewing's sarcoma, is a common side effect of radiation to the bladder. Children require advice, support and encouragement to increase their oral fluid intake. Analgesics and antispasmodics may be of use. Regular monitoring of the urine for blood and infection must be carried out.

Haemopoietic system

Irradiation of the bone marrow, for example the spinal vertebrae in medulloblastoma or CNS leukaemia will decrease the production of the red cells, platelets and leucocytes. Counts will therefore fall as treatment progresses and mild anaemia is not uncommon several months after the completion of treatment.

Regular haematological assays will be required. Patients and parents need to be aware that the white count or platelet level may cause treatment to be temporarily stopped. Haemoglobin levels are generally kept >10 g/dl in order to maintain tumour oxygenation. Hypoxia reduces the effectiveness of irradiation.

The advice given to patients and their families regarding immunosuppression, thrombocytopenia and anaemia are covered in the chemotherapy chapter (6).

Skin

The skin is sensitive to radiation but will normally renew itself in 14–21 days. Acute reactions may occur at the time of treatment or shortly after completion and are usually temporary. When advising children and their parents about skin care there are several important considerations. The area that must be inspected will include the exit site of the beam, not just the entry site. The sensitivity of the skin may be affected by the child's particular skin type, for example whether they burn easily in sunlight, whether the field of irradiation includes skin folds, broken skin or where clothing will rub, for example collars and waistbands, and whether the child is receiving radiosensitizing chemotherapeutic agents, for example actinomycin or doxorubicin.

Skin care programmes are important to minimize the damage caused by the radiation and to relieve symptoms. Individual programmes may differ between centres but the principle should be the same. The area should always be kept clean and dry; gentle washing with unperfumed soap and warm water may be allowed. Drying should be thorough using a soft towel with a patting and blotting action. If the irradiated skin is rubbed harshly or soaps with chemicals are used, there is an increased risk of skin breakdown. Equally, skin that is not dried properly may encourage infection. Generally, skin products such as talcum powder and creams should be avoided (baby products may be allowed) as they may contain chemicals that irritate the skin or metallic elements which may cause scattering of the radiation beams – this in turn may increase the radiation dose to the skin.

Direct heat should be avoided, for example hot water bottles and heat packs, as should direct sunlight. Clothing should be loose fitting, belts and tight collars avoided. Soft or natural fibres may be less irritant and more comfortable. Adhesive dressing tapes should be avoided over the irradiated site.

Acute skin reactions may be: (i) erythema – like sunburn the area becomes pink or red and may tingle; (ii) dry desquamation – the skin is slightly inflamed and becomes dry and scaly. The area may itch and burn and flaking may occur; (iii) moist desquamation – the skin is inflamed and blisters appear. The blisters slough off leaving a denuded area that is painful and exuding serum. Treatment of the above would include re-assessment of the patient's understanding and ability to perform skin care and their compliance. Topical agents, for example hydrocortisone cream 1%, may be prescribed by the radiotherapist. Repeated use of hydrocortisone may cause thinning of the skin and can potentiate superimposed infection, but limited use may help to reduce underlying inflammation. Moist desquamation may require a suspension of treatment, but does not usually cause long-term skin damage.

7.4 BRACHYTHERAPY

In brachytherapy or interstitial therapy the radio-isotope is placed within the tumour or in close proximity, delivering a continuous concentrated dose of radiation. This may be for a few hours or days depending on the strength of the radio-isotope and the dose of radiation.

Occasionally children with soft tissue sarcomas receive brachytherapy using radio-isotopes in a sealed source. The radio-isotope is placed in an applicator and inserted into the body – intracavitary, for example vagina, or interstitial, for example tongue or cheek. Nurses caring for children receiving either of these radioactive isotopes must have an understanding of the fundamental differences. The radio-isotope placed into a body cavity or tissue does not render the patient radioactive. Only if administered intravenously or systemically is the isotope metabolized by the patient thus rendering them radioactive.

Procedures for dealing with emergencies, for example respiratory arrests and accidents, spillage with radioactive sources, must be established prior to the commencement of treatment. Such procedures are described in Pritchard and David (1988).

Specific nursing care will vary depending on the form of therapy used, however the principles of radiation protection remain the same for all treatments using radio-isotopes.

For detailed information about radiation regulations in the UK the reader is referred to HMSO (1985a,b).

To ensure that nurses caring for children receiving sealed or unsealed radioactive treatments receive the lowest dose practical of radiation the following three principles must be adhered to:

1. *Time*. Daily permissible exposure times are calculated according to local rules. This is based on the rationale that the longer one is exposed to radiation the greater the dose that will be absorbed. Nurses must plan their workload prior to entering the restricted area and carry out their work as quickly and efficiently as possible.
2. *Distance*. As radiation spreads out over a greater volume it becomes less intense. By doubling the distance from the source the intensity of radiation absorbed is reduced to one-quarter (Inverse Square Law). It is important, therefore, that nurses utilize as many aids as possible to maintain their distance and reduce exposure, for example the use of a vital signs monitor.
3. *Shielding*. Lead shields or screens will help minimize radiation exposure. Nurses carrying out procedures within the restricted area should always position a lead shield between themselves and the patient.

7.5 FRACTIONATED RADIOTHERAPY

Doses in paediatrics range from as low as 30 Gy in Hodgkin's disease and Wilms' tumour to 60 Gy in Ewing's sarcoma. Fraction size and the time over which treatment is given is a compromise between maximum anti-tumour effect and both early and late toxicity. With hyperfractionated irradiation the dose per fraction is reduced but given more than once a day. These small fractions over a prolonged period will be least toxic. 'Accelerated' irradiation with larger fractions given over a shorter period will be more toxic. Accelerated hyperfractionated schedules involve more than one fraction daily, which allows the same total dose to be given over a shorter period but avoiding the toxicity of larger fraction size that would result with simple acceleration. Moreover, this schedule may be more effective by minimizing the time interval between doses during which tumour cell recovery may occur. The latter schedule is under evaluation in Ewing's sarcoma and rhabdomyosarcoma (Figure 7.2).

7.6 CARE OF THE CHILD RECEIVING ^{131}I METAIODOBENZYLGUANIDINE (^{131}I mIBG)

mIBG is a pharmacological analogue of guanethidine. Neuroblastoma cells and other adrenergic tissue tumours, for example phaeochromo-cytoma, take up mIBG in a similar way to that of noradrenaline. This specific uptake enables irradiation to be 'targetted' into tumour thus avoiding some of the normal organ toxicities described above.

mIBG therapy should be carried out in a purpose-built protected suite and each procedure requires several experienced and well-informed nursing staff.

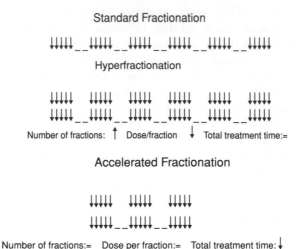

Standard Fractionation

Hyperfractionation

Number of fractions: ↑   Dose/fraction ↓   Total treatment time:=

Accelerated Fractionation

Number of fractions:=   Dose per fraction:=   Total treatment time: ↓

Figure 7.2

Preparation for therapy

Prior to therapy using [131]I mIBG the patient and his family require expert advice, support and guidance to plan for this new form of treatment. The information required will include how the [131]I mIBG is administered, the side effects and restrictions, the length of the isolation period and the role of the parents and other family members. During this interview the ability of the child to comply with the physical and emotional implications of this form of isolation must be assessed. Once the [131]I mIBG is administered the physical contact between the child, his family and hospital personnel is severely restricted. Children who are to comply require careful and sensitive preparation. The playtherapist can help identify activities to promote motivation and prevent anxieties that physical isolation can cause. Decorating the room and creating a homely atmosphere help to make the confinement more bearable.

Children who are unable to comply with the restrictions, either because of their age or developmental status require alternative management. Sedation has proved to be a successful approach but may be required over 2–3 days. Parents of these children require support and comprehensive explanations as to why these measures are necessary.

[131]I mIBG is administered intravenously. A central venous catheter should be inserted to facilitate this and also to avoid the possibility of extravasation of radioactivity during administration, the need for repeated cannulation of a radioactive child and the possible loss of venous access

in the event of an emergency, for example hypertension or respiratory difficulty due to sedation.

Lugol's iodine or potassium iodide is commenced orally two days prior to the administration of the radioactivity and continued for 14 days. The iodine blocks the thyroid, preventing ablation by the radioactive ^{131}iodine. The patient is admitted the day before administration of the ^{131}I mIBG. The central line is checked for patency and the exit site is observed for signs of inflammation or infection. Any dressings are renewed and will be left in position for the period of radioactivity.

The patient's bowel status is also assessed and symptoms of diarrhoea or constipation treated. Diarrhoea is a contamination hazard and constipation inhibits the elimination of radioactivity.

It is advisable that children who are to undergo sedation for the therapy are admitted for a trial of sedation. This ensures that on the day of administration the appropriate drug dosage and timing has been tried and tested. Sedated children will require a nasogastric tube for the administration of further sedation and the Lugol's iodine and a urinary catheter to monitor urine output and minimize contamination of the child and the nurses.

As previously mentioned, ^{131}I mIBG therapy is carried out in a protected room or suite which should include shower and toilet facilities for the patient and a staff area with hand washing facilities. As well as the patient's own preparation of his room the following equipment should also be available: (a) vital signs monitor with variable time setting mode, visible from the staff area, (b) an electronic thermometer, facilitating rapid monitoring of the patient's temperature, and (c) an infusion pump permitting rapid alteration of prescribed infusion rates.

^{131}I mIBG is administered via a battery-operated syringe pump over a period of 30 minutes to 1 hour. The pump is shielded by lead blocks. During the administration transient rise in blood pressure and pulse may occur; these signs are monitored every 5 minutes during the administration, quarter-hourly for the next 4 hours and thereafter as indicated.

All children receiving this therapy will be observed continually for the first 24 hours. Sedated children will be observed continually throughout the sedated period. Nausea is also a side effect of ^{131}I mIBG therapy, especially in the first 24–48 hours. In addition to the psychological reasons, vomiting should be avoided because of the risk of contamination. Knowledge of previously effective anti-emetics is very useful when preparing for ^{131}I mIBG therapy. Children who require sedative anti-emetics may require urinary catheterization for the first 24–48 hours to prevent accidents and contamination.

Prior to the administration the treatment area becomes a restricted zone, the boundary of which is indicated by radiation hazard tape on the floor. Potential contamination areas, for example the toilet floor or the area underneath the urinary drainage system, are protected by wax-backed paper. Radiation warning notices, indicating the amount of time permissible in 24 hours to be spent with the patient, should be displayed prominently.

A ceiling mounted whole body monitor enables the level of radioactivity in the child to be measured and the daily time allowance to be calculated. The amount of time increases as the radioactivity decreases.

To enter the restricted area protective clothing must be donned. This includes plastic overshoes, long sleeve cotton gowns, plastic apron and plastic gloves. Dosimeters and film badges are worn at all times within the treatment area. Once in the treatment area, work is carried out quickly and efficiently. Priority or essential care must be identified and carried out first, leaving basic care for when the permissible time allows.

On leaving the treatment area, overshoes are discarded as the hazard tape is stepped over. This prevents contamination of the floor in the staff area. Plastic aprons are then removed and the gloved hand is checked for levels of contamination. The gloves are then removed carefully to avoid skin contamination and the hands are monitored again. If contaminated, the hands are washed thoroughly until clear of radioactivity. Finally, the gown is removed and checked for contamination using a Geiger counter. If there is no contamination it may be reused.

The patient's personal hygiene is important to prevent recontamination from his or her own body fluids. Boys are requested to sit on the toilet to avoid splashes of urine. The toilet is flushed twice after use. Hands must be washed thoroughly after using the toilet or other possible contact with body fluids, for example brushing of teeth.

Maintaining a good oral intake increases urinary output and increases elimination of radioactivity.

Disposable crockery and cutlery is used and any uneaten food is disposed of in a macerater. Sedated children will receive continuous intravenous fluids to maintain their normal body requirements. All waste, including linen, is stored until decontamination or disposal is carried out by the Physics Department.

As the permissible time with the patient increases, sedated children may be allowed to waken. Parents can be taught the principles of radiation protection and participate in the care of their child to the extent that they are able or wish to do so.

The child will be discharged when the level of radioactivity in their body falls below the legal requirement as set up in the approved code of practice (HMSO, 1985a,b). Details about young children or pregnant relatives will be taken into consideration when planning the discharge. Any contaminated personal effects, for example comforter or soft toys will be stored by the Physics Department until decontaminated.

7.7 CARE OF THE CHILD RECEIVING A SEALED SOURCE OF RADIOACTIVITY

This form of therapy is rarely used in children, however it may be given as part of a combination treatment programme to eradicate a tumour and prevent major surgery. An example of this is vaginal rhabdomyosarcoma, where in order to avoid hysterectomy or sterilization by pelvic irradiation, a caesium or iridium vaginal implant may be used in combination with chemotherapy. With retinoblastoma where in combination with external beam irradiation, plaques of ^{137}Cs or ^{192}Ir are applied to focal areas of the retina. This increases the dose to the 'at risk' area and has a sparing effect on the adjacent tissue (see p. 184). Preparation for this procedure requires expert advice, support and guidance for the patient and her family. Detailed plan of treatment, its indications and side effects must be given with opportunities for questions and discussion.

As before, the patient will be nursed in a protected room with toilet and shower facilities for the patient and hand washing facilities for the staff. The applicator for the sealed source will be made specifically for the patient. This requires a visit to the mould room. To facilitate the making of the mould the patient will require sedation or a light anaesthetic. Once the applicator has been made the patient will be taken to theatre, where it is inserted into the vaginal cavity under general anaesthesia. Perflavin packing may be *in situ* to keep the applicator in position or alternatively the applicator may be stitched into position. The radioactive source is usually loaded into the applicator prior to insertion into the patient. The source remains *in situ* for up to 96 hours. The dose of radiation is lower than that of ^{131}I mIBG therapy but the principles of radiation protection must be adhered to. Time, distance and shielding are still very important. Again, the age and level of development of the patient may necessitate the use of sedation for the procedure. It may be an advantage for the sedated and non-toilet trained patient to be catheterized to prevent soreness in the groin area developing as a result of urine coming into contact with the stitches (if in place). This also reduces the risk of the source falling out when bed pans, potties, are used. The children must remain on bed rest to prevent the source becoming dislodged. A physiotherapist may be involved in creating active passive exercises. As with ^{131}I mIBG therapy, the patient's bowel status is assessed prior to the treatment. A low residue diet is advised during therapy. Sedated children will be hydrated intravenously.

The source should be checked regularly, at least once on each span of duty. The patient should be discouraged from touching the source. A Geiger counter, lead pot and long handle forceps should be positioned near the bed. In the event of the source becoming dislodged or falling out it should be picked up using the long handle forceps (the source should never be handled directly with the fingers) and placed in the lead pot. In this situation, or any other emergency situation, the on-call physicist and radiation protection supervisor should be notified. This is to prevent inadvertent radiation exposure to personnel. All bed linen and waste products are checked with a Geiger counter prior to removal from the environment.

The source will be removed at a predetermined time on the ward by suitably trained nursing staff, following the policy described in Pritchard and David (1988). Unsedated children may require sedation or analgesia such as Entonox to cope with this procedure. It is important that the nurse checks the applicator is intact on removal. Once the source is removed the patient may be discharged within 12–24 hours, depending upon their general condition.

Although the radiation is very localized the patients will require long term follow up, including assessment for scarring or stenosis of the vagina and the opportunity of sexual counselling if required.

7.8 TOTAL BODY IRRADIATION

Total body irradiation (TBI) is used prior to bone marrow transplantation. The role of TBI is threefold (i) to immunosuppress the host, (ii) to make space for the donor marrow – this is not a physical space but an alteration in the microenvironment to facilitate the growth of the transplanted haemopoietic cells, and (iii) antileukaemic or antitumour effect. (Radiation affects non-cycling tumour cells and sanctuary sites such as the testes and central nervous system.)

TBI may be used alone but is more commonly used in combination with cytotoxic drugs such as cyclophosphamide, melphalan, etoposide or cytarabine. It may be given as a single fraction or as fractionated dose given over a number of days, e.g. two fractions at least 6 hours apart for 3 days. Studies comparing single fraction versus fractionated with regard to dose rate effects on normal tissue continue to be evaluated.

Short term side effects include nausea and vomiting, parotitis, erythema, diarrhoea, alopecia, mucositis and bone marrow ablation. Intermediate side effects, occurring 1–3 months post-TBI, include pneumonitis and somnolence. Long term side effects of sterility, endocrine dysfunction, cataracts and second malignancy will be discussed in Chapter 12.

Preparation for this procedure should be included as part of the preparation for bone marrow transplantation. It has been demonstrated that there are three vital elements which enable families to cope through a life-threatening procedure; these are open, honest communication, involvement in the care and ongoing education. The specific preparation for TBI will vary depending upon the age and level of development of the child, his or her previous experience with this form of treatment modality and the relationship between the care team, the patient and the family.

Preparation of the patient includes involvement of the parents who require thorough explanations, verbally and in writing (Ronan and Caserza, 1988). Tape recordings of the explanations and interviews are now becoming more widely used. These give the families opportunity to share and clarify information and does not impose additional stress of parents trying to remember everything that has been said by the doctor or nurse. It also facilitates preparation for the procedures by the parents.

As for external beam irradiation TBI is not an invasive procedure but it does require the patient to lie still, in a room on his or her own. If the patient has received radiotherapy previously the coping mechanisms adopted during that treatment may be of value. However, it must be remembered that even with fractionated TBI each session still takes longer than conventional irradiation. Sedation or general anaesthesia may be required to enable the patient to comply with the 'ordeal' of lying in a room on their own with a large piece of equipment. For fractionated TBI a general anaesthetic may be of preference as sedation twice a day can result in the patient missing out on social activities including meal times.

Test doses are required to measure the distribution of radiation. This provides an opportunity for the patient and his family to meet the staff, observe the room and equipment. Story or music tapes can also be therapeutic during test and treatment periods.

Side effects

Vomiting

Vomiting can occur after a dose of 2–3 Gy has been given to the whole body. The cause of radiation-induced vomiting is not yet fully understood, however experimental data from animal studies suggest that the cause could be irradiation on the upper small bowel causing the release of histamines and prostaglandins or a direct stimulus via the neural pathways from the upper gastrointestinal tract of the chemoreceptor trigger zone. Fasting may help to reduce the incidence of vomiting from this cause. Anxiety and movement have also been identified as having a direct effect on vomiting. Sedation has proved to be a very valuable part of the anti-emetic regimen (Westbrook, Glahome and Barrett, 1987). Knowledge of previous useful anti-emetics is valuable and the addition of dexamethasone and 5-HT$_3$ antagonists has been found to be very effective.

Parotitis

This can occur within 12 hours of the TBI and usually subsides within 48 hours. It can cause severe pain in the jaw which is usually controlled with regular oral analgesia. However, if the pain is severe or if the patient is nauseous and vomiting, intravenous analgesia, e.g. diamorphine, may be required.

Alteration in taste

Alteration in taste due to decreased saliva or thick saliva is not un-common. Dietary advice is covered in Chapter 10.

Erythema

Commonly occurs on days 2–3; it is usually experienced for a short period of time and requires no intervention.

Diarrhoea

Diarrhoea occurs around day 5 and can be a major problem. Accurate monitoring of fluid balance is vital. Antidiarrhoeal agents are of limited use; however regular antispasmodics and analgesics are required for abdominal cramps and pain.

Alopecia

Alopecia begins on or around day 7. It should not be assumed that because the patient has experienced alopecia before they will automatically cope with it again. Psychological preparation concerning altered body image as a result of the transplant should include hair loss and the implications for the patient.

Mucositis

Mucositis will be discussed, as will the supportive care for the pancytopenic patient (Chapter 6).

Somnolence

Patients complain of feeling tired, irritable and lethargic. Pyrexia and anorexia are also quite common. A late somnolent syndrome may occur 6–8 weeks later as with cranial irradiation.

7.9 PALLIATIVE RADIOTHERAPY

The goal of palliative radiotherapy is to relieve symptoms and improve the quality of the child's life. The benefits of the treatment must be carefully measured against the physical and psychological side effects; even at this end stage body image is still very important.

Palliative radiotherapy often involving only a single fraction is a very effective method of relieving bone pain and pain due to pressure or obstruction by tumour. It is also useful in controlling neurological symptoms.

In conclusion, radiotherapy continues to be an important treatment option for children with cancer. However, the recent advances in combination treatment modalities have resulted in the modification of radiotherapy doses and volumes (Tait, 1992). This has resulted in improved survival rates and decreased morbidity.

Paediatric oncology nurses must have an understanding of the different forms of radiation if they are to meet the physical and emotional needs of the child with cancer. When caring for patients receiving brachytherapy they also have responsibility to other patients and colleagues preventing inadvertent exposure to radiation on the ward.

REFERENCES

HMSO (1985a) *The Ionising Radiation Regulations*. HMSO, London.

IIMSO (1985b) *The Protection of Persons against Ionising Radiation arising from any Work Activity*. HMSO, London.

Kun, L.E., Mulhern, R.K. and Criso, J.J. (1983) Quality of life in children treated for brain tumours. *Journal of Neurosurgery*, **58**, 1–6.

Peck, A. and Boland, J. (1977) Emotional reactions to radiation treatment. *Cancer*, **40**, 180–184.

Pritchard, A.P. and David, J. (1988) *Royal Marsden Hospital Manual of Clinical Nursing Policies & Procedures*, Harper & Row, London.

Ronan, J. and Caserza, C. (1988) Development of an educational handbook. Preparing the paediatric patient and family for pre-bone marrow transplant procedures and consultations. *Journal of the Association of Paediatric Oncology Nurses*, **5**(1), 29.

Tait, D. (1992) Minimization and management of morbidity from radiotherapy, in *Paediatric Oncology Clinical Practice and Controversies* (eds P.N. Plowman and C.R. Pinkerton), Chapman and Hall, London, p. 589.

Westbrook, C., Glahome, J. and Barrett, A. (1987) Vomiting associated with whole body irradiation. *Clinical Radiology*, **38**, 263–266.

8 | Bone marrow transplantation

Improved cytotoxic effect may be achieved by dose escalation with administration of very high doses of chemotherapy and radiation. This is only feasible by infusing harvested bone marrow either from the patient himself or a matched donor following treatment. This acts as the 'rescue' reversing permanent or life-threatening myelosuppression (Doney and Buchner, 1985). This procedure is now accepted as standard curative treatment in children with some historically poor prognosis leukaemias and solid tumours. Despite marrow rescue the children undergoing high dose therapy will face potentially life-threatening situations which should not be underestimated in terms of management and support and provides a very challenging and often rewarding aspect of patient care.

Bone marrow transplantation (BMT) is the grafting of bone marrow either from:

1. oneself – autologous BMT
2. a matched donor/another – allogeneic BMT
3. an identical twin – syngeneic BMT

The objective of BMT is to enable administration of high dose chemotherapy with/without total body irradiation at doses otherwise restricted by myelosuppression.

As there are considerable risks with these procedures, the selection of the child depends on the balance of the disease severity against the risk of the procedure (Johnson and Pochedly, 1990; Treleaven and Barrett, 1992). The management of the child receiving autologous or allogeneic BMT is very similar in terms of preparation and administration of the therapy and the monitoring and treating the side effects of myelosuppression. The difference becomes evident when graft versus host disease develops. Consequently, until such time, nursing observation, care and treatment will be described as one.

High dose regimens

A variety of marrow ablative therapies are used prior to the autologous or allogeneic transplant. Deeg *et al.* (1988) describes the objectives of the regimen in allogeneic transplant to be threefold:

1. to create 'room' for the donor grafts to 'take'
2. to immunosuppress the host to allow graft acceptance
3. to eliminate residual malignant disease

The regimens may include single high dose chemotherapeutic agents such as melphalan; a combination of chemotherapeutic agents such as cyclophosphamide or melphalan with busulphan; or a combination of chemotherapy with radiation, such as cyclophosphamide with total body irradiation (Table 8.1). The regimen the child receives depends to a certain degree on local policy; however, diagnosis, age and research protocols may influence the decision.

Tissue typing

Tissue typing is known as the human leucocyte antigen matching (HLA typing). This refers to a series of antigens found on most cells of the body. Antigens are markers on the cell surface that enable recognition by the immune system. The latter recognizes certain HLA types as 'self' but foreign tissue with other HLA is recognized as foreign and a rejection reaction is mounted. If a healthy immunologically competent marrow is HLA matched and transplanted into another, the donor marrow will 'recognize' the matched antigens of the recipient and no rejection will follow. If the donor marrow is insufficiently matched, the donor marrow will recognize the recipient's antigens as foreign and will proceed to mount an immune response against recipient tissue. This response is known as graft versus host disease and can 'be as deadly as the patient's original disease' (Weinberg, 1990) (Figure 8.1).

Table 8.1 Example of high dose therapy regimens used in childhood cancers

Regimen	Disease
Cyclophosphamide–TBI Melphalan–TBI Busulphan–cyclophosphamide	AML ALL
Melphalan Melphalan–carboplatin Busulphan–melphalan–cyclophosphamide	Neuroblastoma Ewing's Rhabdomyosarcoma
BCNU Thiotepa	CNS tumours

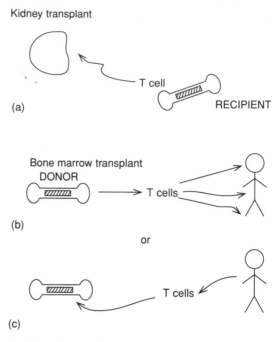

Figure 8.1 (a) Recipient's intact immune system will tend to reject even matched kidney, therefore give cyclosporin to damp down immune response. (b) Recipient immunity ablated by TBI/chemotherapy. Donor T cells will recognize recipient tissue as foreign and 'reject' = GVHD. (c) Some residual recipient immunity may react against donor marrow and cause graft rejection.

Tissue typing involves sampling of blood from family members and the child with the disease. If a sibling appears to have a matched donor (A,B and DR antigens) then a mixed lymphocyte reaction (MLR) is carried out to establish the interaction between the immune system of the donor and recipient. Lymphocytes from the donor are mixed with irradiated lymphocytes from the recipient so that any effect is in one direction and the procedure repeated with irradiated donor cells and recipient lymphocytes. Thus a high MLR between donor and recipient means that the donor cell has recognized HLA types on the surface of the recipient cells and is reacting against it by proliferating. This would predict that *in vivo* GVHD will occur. If the MLR is non-reactive, then a sibling match has been found. Statistically, one in four children has an HLA identical family donor.

Bone marrow harvest

The purpose of a bone marrow harvest is to collect enough stem cells to fully reconstitute the haemopoietic system. The stem cells are able to self-replicate and thus serve as precursor cells to the various blood components, first in the marrow and then in the peripheral blood.

Bone marrow harvesting is carried out under general anaesthetic. The marrow is usually drawn from the iliac crests although occasionally the sternum may need to be used. Regular counts are carried out during the procedure to ensure enough stem cells are collected. The harvested marrow is mixed with heparin to prevent clotting and filtered to remove fat and bone. In general a minimum harvest of 2×10^8 nucleated cells/kg is collected.

If the child has been considered for BMT with minimal residual disease, the marrow may be purged. The purpose of purging is to remove residual tumour cells and involves *in vitro* treatment of the harvested marrow. Chemotherapy may be used to achieve this; the rationale being that tumour cells are more sensitive to chemotherapy than stem cells. However, there is a risk that the healthy stem cells will be affected and engraftment delayed. Moreover, there is no conclusive evidence that purging influences relapse rate. Monoclonal antibodies may be used to target specifically the malignant cells, leaving the other cells unharmed. Physical separation of malignant cells from bone marrow based on density of normal and malignant cells is a third method that has been used.

The timing of the harvest means that some marrow harvests will require cryopreservation. Indications for 'early' harvesting may be a lengthy pre-transplant regimen as marrow should not be left unfrozen for more than 24 hours. Alternatively, in order to avoid stem cell damage after repeated chemotherapy, the harvest may be done early in treatment. Cryopreservation is rarely necessary in allogeneic BMT.

The marrow requiring cryopreservation is frozen to a minimum temperature of $-135°C$ in dimethylsulfoxide (DMSO) which allows safe freezing by maintaining the integrity of the cell membrane (Alessandrino, 1989). Although cryopreserved marrow is usually reinfused within a year, successful reinfusion has been reported up to eight years later.

Peripheral stem cell harvest

Although the bone marrow is the main source of the haemopoietic stem cells, it has been demonstrated that small numbers of stem cells circulate in the peripheral blood and are capable of restoring haematopoiesis after a patient has received megatherapy. It is estimated that 40 aphoresis procedures using a cell separator would be required to restore haematopoiesis under normal circumstances but patients who have received chemotherapy and experience myelosuppression show a marked rise in peripheral stem cell population as the total white count recovers. This is usually 15–20 days after discontinuation of chemotherapy. Consequently if stem cells are collected when the total white count is $1–2 \times 10^9$/l and rising and the platelet count is greater than 50×10^9/l. Fewer procedures are required to achieve marrow reconstitution if GCSF is used.

Peripheral stem cell aphoresis requires a large 'exchange' of blood volume and therefore is not without risk. Two sources of venous access are required, one to remove and one to return blood. A double lumen Hickman catheter is usually not suitable for blood removal due to its flaccidity, and adequate peripheral venous access is required. Cannulation may be distressing to younger children if repeated frequently. Platelets may also be removed due to the similar density of these cells and consequently there may be a drop in the total platelet count.

The number of stem cells transfused is directly correlated with the speed of haemopoietic reconstitution. Infusion of stem cells after marrow ablative therapy has impressively reduced the duration of neutropenia which is reflected in fewer febrile episodes and earlier healing of the gut mucosa. This may therefore decrease the risk of transplant-related early mortality from gram-negative septicaemias and fungaemias.

A bone marrow harvest is usually also frozen in case the stem cells fail to engraft thus providing a 'back-up'. Peripheral stem cell harvests have also been shown to be beneficial when given in conjunction with a bone marrow harvest. Fewer aphoreses are required which is more tolerable in children and the effect of giving both at the same time is an early rise in platelet count and the total white cell count at around day 10, allowing isolation to be terminated. Adjunct peripheral stem cells alone are usually unable to produce sustained engraftment and the total white count may fall again. However, marrow engraftment will occur about this time and thus the overall pancytopenic period reduced.

8.1 PREPARATION FOR BONE MARROW TRANSPLANTATION

Preparation of a child who requires BMT should begin long before a specific date is set. Many parents will be aware that their child is being considered for transplant and they may be acutely aware of the progress of other children undergoing BMT in their own centre. Transplant preparation should result in positive reinforcement for the procedure, but may induce negative feelings with associated anxiety.

Parents will be seen by the consultant oncologist who explains the rationale for the transplant, the specific plan for their child and the potential complications, both short term and long term. Most units provide information which can be taken away, read and discussed with other family members and this is always found to be particularly useful (Ronan and Caserza, 1988). Discussion and question time should be made available with an option to make further appointments to discuss any issues which may subsequently arise. An introduction to a family who have experienced similar circumstances may be beneficial and supportive.

The age of the child is an important consideration when these discussions take place. The older informed child may want to be directly involved in the decision making. They may have great anxieties about how the transplant may affect body image, sexuality/fertility and may have fear of death (particularly if they have experienced the death of a friend following BMT). Sensitivity to these issues is important and a talk with the child on his own is important. Young children and adolescents are sensitive to the parents' feelings and anxieties and often want to protect them from their own worries. Only when all parties have been informed and the full implications of the BMT procedure have been discussed should the transplant proceed.

Family preparation

Bone marrow transplantation is a lengthy procedure, thus before the child is admitted to hospital, much preparation needs to occur to ensure the whole family is ready. It is usually the mother who stays with her sick child, thus separation from her spouse occurs. This must be discussed and grandparents may be able to ensure they have some time out together. Other siblings are a major consideration. Arrangements need to be made so that they can live as normal a life as the circumstances permit. Schooling must be discussed with regard to all siblings. The sick child, if of school age, will be visited by the hospital school teacher and arrangements made for appropriate work to be done whilst in hospital. In the long term, a home tutor may be required and this should be organized in good time for discharge. Other siblings may be experiencing emotions of guilt, fear and neglect which may be manifest in poor attainment at school and behavioral problems, all due to the disruption of 'normal' family life. It is important that the appropriate people are aware of how long the problems may continue. Financial considerations must be addressed. Undoubtedly the financial costs of having a sick child may be vast. The family will be seen by the social worker who will be involved in all these considerations in conjunction with other members of the multidisciplinary team.

Preparation of child

An assessment of the child to determine whether they can tolerate a transplant is necessary. The majority of children will have a break between their last course of chemotherapy and their megatherapy. During this time the child will be seen and monitored by the dietitian to attempt to obtain optimum nutritional status for the procedure. She will provide advice and nutritional supplements if necessary. Rarely the child will need admitting prior to megatherapy for nutritional reasons. The medical examination will ensure that the child is infection-free as far as is detectable. Investigations will also be organized prior to admission; these include:

Full blood count
Ureas + electrolytes
Liver function tests
Clotting screen
Grouping (if not available)
Hepatitis and CMV serology
Other tests depend on local policy but may include HIV, VDRL
Glomerular filtration rate
Chest X-ray
ECG tracing ± echocardiogram
Thyroid function tests

If central venous access is not already *in situ*, this will be carried out under general anaesthetic prior to admission for megatherapy; usually a double or triple lumen line is necessary.

Sibling donors

Sibling donors need special care and attention in preparation for the procedure. Whilst plenty of positive input will be instilled in terms of being 'very special' and a great fuss will be made of them, there may be significant underlying anxiety. Their 'ordeal' may be belittled in terms of comparing it with that of the sick child. The very young child may not be able to understand what is happening, does not feel unwell and therefore cannot understand why they are in hospital. Lengthy explanations using language and play appropriate to the age of the donor is very important. A young child may believe that parents have not told them the truth and that they have the same illness as their sibling. Honesty in terms of the pain and discomfort the donor may experience is vital as many children test adults in terms of honesty and trust them accordingly.

Older sibling donors may have inner conflicts about what is happening. It is often assumed that a sibling will unquestionably want to be their sibling's donor and provide the chance of cure but they may have great fears and genuinely not want to go through with this. Guilt will follow with a reluctance to discuss these feelings.

If the patient dies as a result of the BMT procedure, sibling donors may have great difficulty in coming to terms with the death. Long-term psychological effects may be devastating and require long-term follow up and counselling as appropriate.

Work-up towards being a bone marrow donor (HLA typing having been established) will include a visit to the out-patient department and the ward if unfamiliar to the donor. An explanation of exactly what will happen should be given. The donor will need to have a series of blood tests very similar to their brother/sister as well as a chest X-ray and ECG. The medical and anaesthetic staff need to examine the donor and to take a medical history to ensure they are fit enough for an anaesthetic.

The donor is usually admitted to the ward the day before the harvest and transplant is to take place. Routine preoperative preparation will be carried out. The donor usually requires a blood transfusion postoperatively. If appropriate to age and the child consents, this may be autologous and taken from the donor 10–14 days previously. It must be ensured whether autologous or donated that the blood is available prior to theatre. Few, if any, adverse effects to the donor from the harvest procedure have been reported, although fat embolism has been described as an extremely rare complication. The donor is usually discharged the following day with adequate pain control. However, many children recover extremely quickly, are mobile without discomfort and are discharged on the same day.

Marrow ablative therapy

Some of the commoner high dose regimens are described in Table 8.1. The paediatric oncologist (medical or nursing) responsible for administering the prescribed drugs must be aware of the potential immediate side effects and the rationale for the manner in which the regimen has been prescribed. Accurate documentation of all drugs given is imperative for safe 24-hour care of these children. TBI is detailed in Chapter 7.

Reinfusion of bone marrow/stem cells

The timing of the marrow reinfusion will depend on the high-dose regimen. Melphalan, for example is eliminated within 12 hours whereas etoposide metabolites take up to 72 hours. Fresh marrow should be infused as soon as possible after harvest, although up to 48 hours marrow remains viable. Infusion of fresh autologous marrow will present no problems in terms of sensitivity reactions but its volume may require a diuretic cover to maintain fluid balance.

Allogeneic marrow presents problems as with any other blood product and some centres routinely premedicate with hydrocortisone and Piriton. Again a diuretic may be required to maintain balance particularly if the donor is a teenager and the recipient a toddler. Cryopreserved marrow and stem cells pose the problem of reactions to the preservative (DMSO) used in freezing the marrow. Potential complications include hypersensitivity to the DMSO with haemodynamic instability. Anaphylaxis, although extremely rare, has been reported. More commonly, an immediate taste often described as 'sweetcorn' causes nausea and vomiting and may last 24–48 hours. Other reported reactions include headache, abdominal cramps, lightness of the chest, hypertension, hypotension and raised liver function tests. These side effects can be minimized and, for many, eliminated with hyperhydration and a premedication of hydrocortisone, chlorpheniramine and a small dose of pethidine.

Haemoglobinuria is seen in some children and manifests itself in red urine. Probably the most important nursing action is to warn the family as this can be extremely frightening. Hyperhydration commenced several hours prior to infusion of the marrow and continued until the urine is clear of haemoglobin will help prevent occlusion of the renal tubules. A diuretic may be required to maintain fluid balance.

Isolation

Bone marrow transplantation necessitates a period of physical isolation as the total white blood count falls below $0.5 \times 10^9/l$ for a considerable length of time. Methods such as laminar air flow (LAF), high efficiency particulate air filtration (HEPA) and reverse barrier nursing are all still used in an attempt to minimize the risk of exogenous infection. The fact that these techniques vary widely between centres suggests the need for research into these methods to determine whether one method is more effective than another. Some units also use gut decontamination with antibiotics such as colistin and neomycin and sterile food and water to minimize the occurrence of endogenous septicaemias. The effectiveness of this also needs further evaluation. Dezenhall (1987) studied nutritional support in BMT patients and reported that sterile diet was rarely used due to poor tolerance. Paediatric patients find the antibiotics intolerable and difficult to swallow during the phase of severe mucositis. Studies to date regarding the isolation technique appear to conclude that there is no difference in survival rates between simple reverse barrier nursing and the more elaborate techniques (Armstrong, 1984; Bodey, 1984).

Inadequately handwashed and dried hands are a known source of cross-infection (Garner & Ferrero, 1986; Larson, 1985) which is borne out in many studies which show that the single most important factor in prevention of infection is effective handwashing.

The Infection Control Nurses Association reported on the use of protective clothing in prevention of cross-infection. Whilst most of their work was not in the oncological setting much can be learnt from these studies. Transfer of infection from uniforms was evaluated and considered significant regardless of fabric. Such infection was mostly preventable with the use of plastic aprons. Changing of aprons is important and must be carried out for each patient or more often if the apron becomes wet through nursing duties.

BMT units appear to be tending towards reverse barrier isolation methods with varying degrees of 'gowning-up' and emphasis on hand-washing. The use of simpler methods of isolation is supported by the fact that with the number of broad-spectrum antibiotic cover available, death from bacterial infection has diminished considerably.

The timing of commencement of isolation varies according to local policy. Some units admit the child directly into isolation whilst others wait until after radiation therapy (isolation needs to be broken for this pro-cedure). For those children who are not receiving radiation treatment, isolation may be delayed until the total white blood count falls below $1 \times 10^9/l$. There is no literature available to support any of the above strategies.

Isolation is generally discontinued when the neutrophil count is con-sistently greater than $0.5 \times 10^9/l$ and rising. Obviously common sense precautions need to continue as the child may not be ready for discharge at this point. At busier visiting times and out-patient clinics the child may benefit from staying in their room.

The side effects of chemotherapeutic drugs are described in Chapter 6. Nursing care and observations specific to BMT will be detailed here.

Psychosocial care of child in isolation

Most of the child's preparation for his BMT will have occurred in the out-patient department. Although the mother usually resides with the child, she may change with her husband at the weekends; this will provide three functions: the father will not feel excluded from what is happening to his child; the mother can spend time with other siblings and the mother can have time out from the intensity of the hospital situation. The family will be advised to come prepared with plenty to occupy their child. Most BMT rooms provide a T.V., video and telephone. However, computer games, favourite toys, posters to decorate the room and make it more homely should be encouraged.

The majority of paediatric units have a family-centred philosophy to patient care, creating a stimulating and supportive environment for the child. Parents are encouraged with guidance and support to assume the role of primary care giver. The nurse must, however, be sensitive to parents' feelings and emotions and may need to provide some aspects of the child's care on a temporary basis. An example of this is mouth care which may be painful due to mucositis and the parents may feel unable to insist their child carries out this painful procedure. The nurse will need to take over leaving mum to provide cuddles afterwards.

At times the care-giving parent will need to take a break and this time must be planned into the child's individual care plan. Stress levels will rise and a sense of failure and inadequacy will set in if 'time-out' is not given.

Play

When the child is well occupation becomes essential to relieve boredom and frustration and the play therapist has an important role. Play is also a means by which young children learn, cope with stress around them and is a vital part of normal socialization. The aim of play for transplant patients is to provide normal life experiences and to maintain the developmental, cognitive, social and emotional health of the child (Axline, 1969). It is important to maintain this throughout hospitalization. If the play therapist does not know the child who is to undergo BMT the pretransplant period will be used to observe the child's likes, dislikes, interests and coping strategies.

Throughout the isolation period the play therapist should maintain contact on a daily basis. The child may be too sick to play but sitting with the child, reading to them or leaving a toy that they may play with later, ensures the child does not feel abandoned at their most sick time (Petrillo and Sanger, 1980). The fact that the specialist still maintains contact with the child when they are extremely ill is interpreted by children as evidence that they are expected to recover.

The play therapist is obviously unable to play with one child all day and she therefore needs to involve parents in hospital play. When a child is sick in hospital, parents are under great stress and need support and the parents may not appreciate that play is a vital part of child development enabling the learning of new skills and dealing with stress and experiences. Parents know their child's feelings and frustrations better than anyone else and can observe him accordingly. The parent can then be ready with extra encouragement and stimulating ideas when the child is ready, preventing apathy in the child which is all too often seen.

Parents can work closely with the play therapist communicating their observations and/or fears and be advised and helped by provision of appropriate activity. When the therapist is able to sit or play with their child, the parent can safely leave their child confidently knowing that he is not about to have any painful procedure carried out and the parent can enjoy her 'time-out'.

Schooling

Schooling, as mentioned will have to be planned for even before the transplant procedure has begun. The teacher, if the child is of school age, should continue to encourage the child's schooling, as the medical condition dictates. School friends are a vital part of the child's life and continual contact should be encouraged. Cards, letters, telephone calls and if possible a tape are all positive ways to let the child know he/she has not been forgotten. Conversely, the school friends need regular update on their friend's condition and progress.

Physiotherapy

Whilst a child is isolated and in a limited space, there is a tendency to stay on the bed. Physiotherapy, especially if the unit is fortunate enough to have its own physiotherapist, can play an important part in preventing muscle weakness, maintaining a sense of well-being and can also be fun. The child, if possible, should be seen daily and an exercise plan developed to include arms, legs and chest exercises. As the child's condition dictates, active exercises may need to be taken over and carried out passively. The physiotherapists can work with parents and teach them the routine and tick charts put on the wall. The exercises can be carried out several times a day and the physiotherapist can visually see how well the child is doing. Exercise bicycles are fun and can be put in the isolation rooms. Mums can do some exercises as well!

When isolation is terminated, a visit to the physiotherapy department for short periods continues to strengthen the physical status of the child. The nurse and physiotherapist work closely together to arrange a time when the department will be free for a BMT patient only, and when intravenous administration is either simple fluids or temporarily discontinued.

8.2 GRAFT VERSUS HOST DISEASE

Graft versus host disease (GVHD) is a common complication of allogeneic transplants. It is the complication whereby the donor marrow, which has largely replaced the recipient's immune system, identifies foreign antigens in the recipient and responds by manifesting an immune response (Figures 8.1, 8.2) GVHD results when the donor T-lymphocytes reject the tissue of the bone marrow recipient.

The incidence of GVHD in HLA identical siblings is reported to be approximately 45% (Storb et al., 1985; Bortin et al., 1989). GVHD may become evident between 10–80 days after BMT and may be very mild or become life threatening (McDonald, 1986). The disease targets three main organs, the skin, the gastrointestinal tract and the liver, although any organ can be involved.

It is unclear why GVHD develops in some patients and not in others despite prophylactic T-lymphocyte suppression using methotrexate or

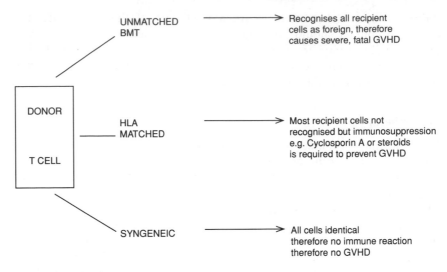

Figure 8.2 Effect of donor T cell population.

cyclosporin A. However, some risk factors have become apparent which include a sex mismatch BMT (particularly a female donor to a male recipient), the number of blood product transfusions and the age of the patient (older age are more at risk) (Bortin *et al.*, 1989; Weisdorf *et al.*, 1990).

Graft versus host disease occurring within 3 months is referred to as acute graft versus host disease and beyond this, chronic graft versus host disease (Graze and Gale, 1979).

The three organs targetted will be described and the nursing implications detailed individually.

Skin graft versus host disease

A skin rash is usually the first manifestation of graft versus host disease. It usually appears as an erythematous rash on the soles of the feet, palms of the hands, cheeks and ears. This may develop into a red papular lichen planus rash over the whole body. If untreated this may develop into severe erythema and wet desquamation and blistering may follow. The superficial layers of the skin may slough away and hyper- or hypopigmentation becomes evident.

If this is untreated or unresponsive to treatment, the skin may lose its elasticity, ulceration may occur and contractures develop.

Nursing implications

The aim is to maintain the integrity of the skin to promote patient comfort and prevent infection. A daily lukewarm bath using oil in the water is soothing. The skin should be patted dry (not rubbed). A moisturizing cream will prevent drying and cracking of the skin, maintain the skin integrity and help prevent access for secondary infection. Cream should be applied liberally at least twice daily and more often if necessary. The skin in these children is very sensitive to temperature changes and the child may become cold quite quickly. Planning and organizing of the bath is important in terms of efficiency and speed.

Soaps, if preferred on discharge, should be non-irritant and not highly perfumed. Baby soap is recommended.

Cotton clothing which is loose is recommended to help any associated irritation and pruritus although antihistamines may be required.

If any lesions develop into blisters, these lesions need to be as carefully treated as burns with appropriate creams, for example Flamazine helps prevent *Pseudomonas* infection. The child may need to be on foam which will absorb any exudate from burst blisters and is comfortable.

Skin care as outlined will continue until otherwise advised in the outpatient department. Protection of the skin from the sun is important. Anders and Leach (1983) advise that protection from sunlight using high factor protection should continue for at least a year.

Secondary infection is a potential complication and therefore continuous observation of the skin carried out. Any suspicious areas should be swabbed and sent for culture and regular observations of temperature, pulse and blood pressure taken with abnormal results reported immediately.

Nutritional considerations

Nutritional considerations become more evident in severe skin GVHD when energy and protein requirements may be considerable; if more than 50% of the body is involved protein needs and fluid loss may increase. Weight and accurate fluid balance chart are important and the dietitian can advise on replacement of protein. Biochemistry will be reviewed as the child's condition dictates and if necessary replaced intravenously. Parenteral nutrition, in severe cases, may need to be considered.

Physiotherapy

Physiotherapy will be extremely important as the skin may be painful and sore and the child may be reluctant to mobilize. Loss of elasticity of the skin may be preventable and this is essential to avoid contractures.

Gastro-intestinal tract graft versus host disease

This usually presents as green watery diarrhoea, the volume corresponding to the extent of the mucosal damage (Wolford and McDonald, 1988). The diarrhoea consists of mucus, protein, cellular debris and is often occult blood positive on testing. Protein content is high and this is reflected in falling plasma protein levels.

The child will experience spasmodic crampy abdominal pains which are usually relieved partially or wholly on passing a stool. There may be associated nausea and vomiting. The volume of diarrhoea may range from 500 ml to several litres.

Nursing implications

The objective of care for the child with gut GVHD is to promote patient comfort and maintain fluid and electrolyte balance.

The child with severe diarrhoea may become dehydrated and sick very quickly. Maintenance of strict fluid balance is imperative which includes, when possible, the volume of diarrhoea and urine separately.

Associated abdominal pain, nausea and vomiting may respond to anti-emetics and antispasmodics and these should be tried to promote patient comfort. The child's weight should be monitored at least daily. Blood biochemistry will be monitored as the child's condition dictates and may be several times a day. Potassium loss can be great, as will protein loss and these will need correcting. The volume and nature of fluid replacement will depend on the extent of volume loss and plasma electrolytes. Antidiarrhoeals such as loperamide may be of value.

Desquamation of the gut lining may occur and parents should be warned of this as it can be very frightening. The child may still be thrombocytopenic with a risk of haemorrhage. Platelet counts will be reviewed frequently and in the event of melaena may be supported at a higher than normal level to keep the level above $50 \times 10^9/l$ in an attempt to prevent major haemorrhage.

Attention to the child's perianal region is important. The area should be washed in warm oily water and patted dry to help maintain its integrity and prevent excoriation. Liberal application of barrier cream is advised.

If GVHD prophylaxis, e.g. cyclosporin, has been via the oral route, this will need to be changed to the intravenous route.

Nutritional considerations

Gastrointestinal tract GVHD usually necessitates parenteral nutrition to aid gut healing by providing complete rest, and supporting the child's nutritional requirements. Limiting oral intake will reduce the volume of diarrhoea (Wolford and McDonald, 1988) which includes disallowing even sips of water. As diarrhoea settles and the GI tract has had healing time, diet can be introduced very slowly and TPN titrated to meet the child's nutritional needs, as advised by the dietitian.

Liver graft versus host disease

Liver GVHD usually presents with raised liver enzymes. The child may also complain of right upper quadrant pain and have hepatomegaly on examination (Ford and Ballard, 1988). Jaundice usually develops as the disease progresses. In severe liver GVHD, ascites and ultimately encephalopathy may develop.

Nursing implications

Nursing care is aimed at supportive treatments and comfort of the child. Analgesia may be required and anti-emetics if nausea is apparent. Pruritus due to jaundice may cause itching and antihistamines may be required.

Coagulation may be affected due to disruption of normal liver function. Daily clotting screens should be taken and clotting factors given as required.

If severe liver GVHD ensues with associated ascites and encephalopathy all supportive care will be given to promote comfort as the disease is invariably fatal at this stage.

Nutritional considerations

Parenteral nutrition is usually required in patients with liver GVHD. However, the use of lipids in these patients is controversial, and close observation of liver function will be carried out. Lipids may be discontinued to see whether liver function is affected.

Treatment of graft versus host disease

Cyclosporin A (CSA) and intravenous methotrexate are long established drugs used in the prevention of GVHD. The treatment of GVHD has been studied at length in terms of the use of single agent versus multiple agents and drug toxicity. Storb *et al.* (1985) compared CSA against methotrexate as single agent prophylaxis and although each causes different side effects which are problematic, survivorship of these patients was similar.

With the combination of CSA and methotrexate survival was improved (Deeg *et al.*, 1982; Storb *et al.*, 1986) with the incidence of GVHD reduced and thus fewer incidences of associated fatal infections.

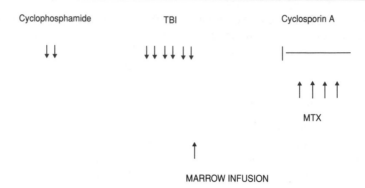

Figure 8.3 A commonly used allograft regimen including the 'Seattle' GVHD prophylaxis protocol.

To date, this combination is the preferred prophylactic treatment for GVHD. CSA is commenced the day prior to the transplant and given intravenously twice daily until gastrointestinal toxicity has resolved and the child can tolerate the oral preparation. Methotrexate is given intravenously on days 1, 3, 6 and 11 (Figure 8.3). A major side effect of this is mucositis exacerbating the mucositic effects of the high dose chemotherapy and radiation. Folinic acid rescue given at 24 hours for one day after each methotrexate dose may help reduce this.

Despite prophylaxis, GVHD occurs and its standard treatment is high dose steroids. The course of this depends on the course of the GVHD. Other drugs such as azathioprine and thalidomide have been evaluated and found to be effective. Research continues to be directed towards the use of other T-cell suppressors as well as current drugs to determine the optimum drug with the least toxicity. GVHD continues to be a great challenge to oncology specialists, and specialist nurses should be aware of early signs of GVHD and be knowledgeable regarding drug treatment and associated side effects.

Graft versus leukaemia effect

Studies of long-term survivors of allogeneic bone marrow transplantation suggest that those patients who experience GVHD are less likely to relapse than those who do not. Those patients with GVHD II–IV, have a relapse rate 2–5 times lower than syngeneic BMT or those allogeneic BMT patients who did not experience GVHD (Weiden *et al.*, 1979).

It should be mentioned that GVHD can be almost abolished by removing T cells from the donor marrow. This 'T-cell depletion' is achieved by incubating the marrow with anti-T cell monoclonal antibodies which selectively lyse the T cells which produce GVHD. Unfortunately this may have an adverse effect on marrow reconstitution and moreover reduces the beneficial graft versus leukaemia effect which occurs in parallel with GVHD (Martin *et al.*, 1985; Mitsuyasu, 1986). In children, as opposed to adults, T-cell depletion is generally restricted to mismatched BMT or matched unrelated donor (MUD) transplants where GVHD morbidity is high.

Haematological support

Haematological support is discussed in the chapter on chemotherapy and therefore only support specific to BMT will be discussed here.

Irradiated blood products

The transfusion of blood products in the immunocompromised patient has the potential to cause GVHD. Lymphocytes within the blood product may engraft and mount an immune response and graft versus host disease may result. By irradiating blood products with 15–25 Gy, the proliferative ability of the lymphocytes is terminated and engraftment cannot take place.

Cytomegalovirus (CMV)

CMV is a major cause of morbidity and death in BMT patients Treatment of established disease is very difficult although ganciclovir combined with CMV hyperimmune immunoglobulin may be effective. Blood products which are CMV positive may pose a problem to severely immunocompromised BMT patients who are CMV seronegative. Consequently, it is practice to determine the child's CMV status prior to BMT and if he is seronegative, seronegative blood products given to minimize the risk of a CMV pneumonitis developing. Any child who is likely to have a BMT, e.g. AML, high count ALL, t9;22 all should receive CMV-negative products unless shown to already be CMV seropositive. Where either donor or recipient are CMV positive, prophylaxis using high-dose acyclovir or ganciclovir has been advocated.

REFERENCES

Alessandrino, E.P. (1989) Cryopreservation of marrow cells for ABMT. Is there any effect on the harvested leukaemic cells? *Bone Marrow Transplantation*, **(S4)**, 81–84.

Anders, J.E. and Leach, E.E. (1983) Sun versus skin. *American Journal of Nursing*, **83**, 1015–1020.

Armstrong, D. (1984) Protected environments are discomforting and expensive and do not offer meaningful protection. *American Journal of Medicine*, **76**, 685–689.

Axline, V. (1969) In *Play Therapy*, Ballantine, New York.

Bodey, G. (1984) Current status of prophylaxis of infection with protected environments. *American Journal of Medicine*, **76**, 678–684.

Bortin, M.M., Atkinson, K., van Kekkum, DW. *et al*. (1989) Factors influencing the risk of acute and chronic GVHD in humans. A preliminary report from the IBMTR. *Bone Marrow Transplantation*, **4**, S(1) 222–224.

Deeg, H.J., Klingemann, H., Phillips, G. *et al*. (1988) *A Guide to Bone Marrow Transplantation*, Springer Verlag, New York.

Deeg, H.J., Storb, R., Weiden, PL. *et al*. (1982) Cyclosporin A and methotrexate in canine marrow transplantation engraftment. Graft versus host disease and induction of tolerance. *Transplantation*, **34**, 30–35.

Dezenhall, A. (1987) Food and nutrition services in BMT centers. *Journal of the American Dietetic Association*, **87**, 1351–1353.

Doney, K. and Buchner, C. (1985) Bone marrow transplantation overview. *Plasma Therapy Transfusion Technology*, **6**, 149–161.

Ford, R. and Ballard, B. (1988) Acute complications after BMT. *Seminars in Oncology Nursing*, **4**(1), 15–24.

Garner, J.S. and Ferrero, M.S. (1986) Handwashing and hospital environmental control. *American Journal of Infection Control*, **14**(3), 110–129.

Graze, P.R. and Gale, G.P. (1979) Chronic GVHD: A syndrome of disordered immunity. *American Journal of Medicine*, **66**, 611–620.

Johnson, F.L. and Pochedly, C. (1990) *Bone Marrow Transplantation in Children*, Raven Press, New York.

Larson, E. (1985) Handwashing and skin. *American Journal of Infection Control*, **6**(1), 14–83.

McDonald, G.B. (1986) Intestinal and hepatic complications of human BMT (Parts I and II). *Gastroenterology*, **90**, 460–477.

Martin, P.J., Hansen, J.A., Buckner, C.D. *et al*. (1985) Effects of *in vitro* depletion of T-cells in HLA identical allogeneic marrow grafts. *Blood*, **66**, 664.

Mitsuyasu, R.T. (1986) Treatment of donor bone marrow with monoclonal anti-T-cell antibody and complement for the prevention of GVHD. *ANNALS International of Medicine*, **105**, 29.

Petrillo, M. and Sanger, S. (1980) *Emotional Care of Hospitalized Children*, Lippincott, Philadelphia.

Ronan, J. and Caserza, C. (1988) Development of an educational handbook. Preparing the paediatric patient and family for pre-bone marrow transplant procedures and consultations. *Journal of the Association of Paediatric Oncology Nurses*, **5**(1), 4–13.

Storb, R., Deeg, H.J., Thomas, E.D. *et al*. (1985) Marrow transplantation for chronic myelocytic leukaemia. A controlled trial of cyclosporin versus methotrexate for prophylaxis of graft versus host disease. *Blood*, **66**, 698–702.

Storb, R., Deeg, J.H., Whitehead, J. *et al*. (1986) Methotrexate and cyclosporin compared with cyclosporin alone for prophylaxis of acute graft versus host disease after marrow transplantation for leukaemia. *New England Journal of Medicine*, **314**(12), 729–735.

Treleaven, J. and Barrett J. (1992) *Bone Marrow Transplantation in Practice*, Churchill Livingstone, Edinburgh.

Weiden, P., Flournoy, N., Donnall Thomas, E. *et al.* (1979) Anti-leukaemic effect of GVHD in human recipients of allogeneic marrow grafts. *New England Journal of Medicine*, **300**, 1068–1073.

Weinberg, P. (1990) The human leukocyte antigen (HLA) system, the search for a matching donor. National marrow donor programme development and marrow donor issues, in *BMT Principles, Practice and Nursing Insights*, Marie, Bakitus, Whedon (5), 105–131.

Weisdorf, D., Haake, R., Blazar, B. *et al.* (1990) Treatment of moderate/severe acute graft versus host disease after allogeneic bone marrow transplantation: An analysis of clinical risk features and outcome. *Blood*, **75**(4), 1024–1030.

Wolford, J.L. and McDonald, G.B. (1988) A problem orientated approach to intestinal and liver disease after marrow transplantation. *Journal of Clinical Gastroenterology*, **10**, 419–433.

9 | Individual tumours

9.1 THE LEUKAEMIAS

Leukaemia is the malignant transformation of haemopoietic precursor cells in the bone marrow. The stage at which this transformation occurs determines the lineage involved and thus the characteristics of the leukaemic cell clone. Sub-classification is based on the clinical behaviour of the disease, i.e. acute or chronic, and on the cell lineage, i.e. myeloblastic, lymphoblastic, megakaryocytic and erythroblastic. Finally, with lymphoblastic and myelocytic leukaemias there are further sub-groups determined by morphological features – FAB classification (Bennett, Catovsky and Daniel, 1976), cytochemical staining and immunological surface markers. The latter are antigens on cell membrane or in cytoplasm which can be detected by immunofluorescence techniques using monoclonal antibodies raised against these antigens (Table 9.1). These surface antigens are described by CD (cluster differentiation) numbers, e.g. CD10 common ALL; CD19, 20 B lineage; CD2, 4 T lineage; CD13 myeloid lineage.

Aetiological factors in leukaemia remain obscure. A transmissible virus has been demonstrated in feline leukaemia and the retrovirus HTLV 1 is associated with hairy cell leukaemia in man. However, despite speculation, no viral agent has been implicated in childhood leukaemia (Alexander, 1993). Environmental factors remain speculative, e.g. clustering at the site of nuclear generating plants, nuclear disposal sites or high tension electricity installations continues. Paternal radiation exposure has been postulated. Because of the relative rarity of leukaemia in childhood it is difficult to obtain statistically meaningful data on such matters (Craft, Openshaw and Birch, 1984; Gardner *et al.*, 1990). Spontaneous mutation in the actively dividing lymphocyte population, perhaps driven by viral exposure, has been suggested as a causal factor (Greaves and Chan, 1986).

Table 9.1 Classification of leukaemias

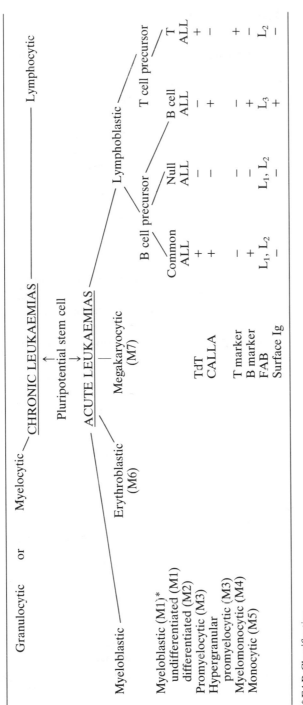

Granulocytic   or   Myelocytic ——— CHRONIC LEUKAEMIAS ——— Lymphocytic

Pluripotential stem cell

ACUTE LEUKAEMIAS ——— Lymphoblastic

Myeloblastic — Myeloblastic (M1)*
undifferentiated (M1)
differentiated (M2)
Promyelocytic (M3)
Hypergranular promyelocytic (M3)
Myelomonocytic (M4)
Monocytic (M5)

Erythroblastic (M6)

Megakaryocytic (M7)

| | B cell precursor | | | T cell precursor |
	Common ALL	Null ALL	B cell ALL	T ALL
TdT	+	-	-	+
CALLA	+	-	+	-
T marker	-	-	-	+
B marker	+	-	+	-
FAB	L_1, L_2	L_1, L_2	L_3	L_2
Surface Ig	-	-	+	-

* FAB Classification

Acute lymphoblastic leukaemia

The suppression of normal myelopoiesis due to marrow infiltration or the involvement of lymph nodes are reflected in the presenting features of acute lymphoblastic leukaemia (ALL). Symptoms may be subtle and resemble other common disorders (Table 9.2). In some patients the diagnosis can be made by examination of the peripheral blood film which contains circulating leukaemic blast cells. A bone marrow aspirate is required for confirmation of diagnosis and sub-classification. Standard cytochemical and immunological tests currently done are shown in Table 9.3. Occasionally transient marrow hypoplasia precedes ALL and may mimic aplastic anaemia as may reactive lymphocytosis due to viral infections. Other clinical signs are usually helpful. If in doubt it is advisable to repeat the marrow aspirate at a later date as the disease will eventually declare itself. Spinal fluid is normally examined at presentation, although if the peripheral blast cell count is very high this may be delayed for several days to avoid the theoretical risk of contaminating the central nervous system with blast cells. Also, to avoid confusion in the interpretation in the event of a traumatic tap. It is unlikely that CSF cytology will be significantly altered by initial chemotherapy and mask disease that was present at diagnosis.

Chest X-rays should be performed routinely to determine if there is mediastinal enlargement which may produce significant tracheal compression in the case of T-cell leukaemia. Abdominal ultrasound is recommended to exclude infiltration of the kidneys, particularly in patients with high presenting white cell count, to avoid renal complications during induction.

The aim of initial treatment in ALL is to achieve remission with intensive chemotherapy. At the end of this 'induction' period the bone

Table 9.2 Childhood disorders presenting with features similar to acute leukaemia

Presenting features	Differential diagnosis
Anaemia, general malaise	Nutritional anaemia, aplastic anaemia, viral illness
Bone and/or joint pain	Rheumatoid arthritis, septic arthritis, osteomyelitis, irritable hip, osteochondritis
Easy bruising	Constitutional, trauma, non-accidental injury, idiopathic thrombocytopenia, aplastic anaemia
Lymphadenopathy	Bacterial infection, mumps, infectious mononucleosis
Liver and spleen enlargement	Viral infection

Table 9.3 Routine evaluation of bone marrow and CSF in suspected leukaemia

Single aspirate

If difficult aspirate or if aplastic anaemia, myelodysplasia or metastatic disease suspected – trephine biopsy should be done

Morphology – On aspirate and/or trephine 'touch prep'
            – Multiple aspirates should be done if 'suspicious' cells seen on single sample

Cytochemistry
– Acid phosphatase – (+ T ALL)
– Periodic acid–Schiff – (+ ALL)
– Sudan black – (+ AML)

FAB classification

Immunological markers
– B, T, or myeloid lineage CD number, TdT (terminal deoxynucleotidyl transferase)
– Surface Ig, cytoplasmic μ

Blast cell karyotype

Gene rearrangement studies – Immunoglobulin gene
                               – T cell receptor gene

CSF tap

Cell count

Cytospin examination

? TdT/immune markers for 'suspicious' cells

marrow should be clear of all detectable disease. Most regimens include vincristine, prednisolone, asparaginase ± daunorubicin (Table 9.4). It is during this period that the maximum morbidity occurs with a significant number of deaths from infections. In patients with bulky disease, i.e. massive lymphadenopathy, liver and spleen involvement or white cell count over $100 \times 10^9/l$, careful attention must be given to electrolyte imbalance and renal function due to the risk of tumour lysis syndrome (Chapter 10). Intensive supportive care may be required and the patient should remain in hospital until the blood count has recovered.

After achieving remission further intensive chemotherapy has been shown to improve survival. High-dose pulsed therapy causing severe transient marrow suppression or a more sustained administration of chemotherapy leading to protracted but less severe myelosuppression is used. Such intensification regimens generally contain additional drugs (Pinkerton *et al.*, 1987), the rationale being that the residual leukaemic population which is resistant to the initial chemotherapy may not be resistant to these drugs.

Table 9.4 Phases of treatment for acute childhood leukaemias (UK regimens)

Type of leukaemia	Induction	CNS-directed treatment	Consolidation	Continuation
Acute lymphoblastic	vincristine prednisolone asparaginase ± daunorubicin	cranial irradiation or intrathecal methotrexate high dose i.v. methotrexate	cytarabine etoposide thioguanine daunorubicin	methotrexate 6-mercaptopurine vincristine prednisolone
Acute myeloblastic	daunorubicin cytarabine thioguanine etoposide amsacrine	intrathecal methotrexate ± cytarabine	repeat induction-type combination or high-dose chemoradiotherapy with bone marrow rescue	

The second phase of treatment is directed toward the central nervous system. Up to 60% of patients relapsed in the central nervous system prior to the development of 'prophylactic' or CNS-directed therapy. Cranial irradiation (18–24 Gy) with several injections of intrathecal methotrexate reduces the incidence of CNS relapse to less than 10%. Concern about the endocrine effects of irradiation, such as growth hormone deficiency and premature puberty, and the adverse effects on intellectual development have led to attempts to rely or chemotherapy alone. This consists of more intensive and prolonged intrathecal chemotherapy, either with methotrexate alone or combined with cytosine arabinoside and hydrocortisone. High-dose intravenous methotrexate will effectively penetrate the central nervous system. Such an approach is probably equally effective for low-risk patients, but this remains to be proven in other groups (Chessells, 1985).

The third phase of treatment is 'maintenance' or 'continuing therapy'. This consists of out-patient treatment with oral drugs and pulses of intravenous chemotherapy, generally continued for two years. The duration of continuing treatment has been progressively reduced. Randomized studies have shown no advantage from more prolonged treatment. In the context of more intensive initial treatment it is conceivable that the duration could be further reduced in the future. During continuing treatment, the patient is immunosuppressed to a significant degree and there is an important risk from *Pneumocystis carinii* and viral infections such as chicken pox and measles. To prevent the former, prophylactic Septrin is given throughout the period of treatment and for the latter immunoglobulin is given after exposure. Acyclovir should be given without hesitation in varicella and zoster infections.

The intensity of treatment influences prognostic features in ALL, but in general adverse factors include age less than one or more than 10 years, male sex, presenting count greater than $20 \times 10^9/l$, L2 morphology, central nervous system leukaemia at presentation and persistence of blast cells in the marrow aspirate two weeks into induction treatment. In the past the B ALL subtype has done very badly on standard regimens, but the outlook has been improved by the use of intensive non-Hodgkin's lymphoma-type regimens. The hypodiploid chromosome karyotype and specific abnormalities such as Ph chromosome t(9;22) or t(4;11) are associated with a poor prognosis.

It is now possible to identify high-risk patients for whom experimental regimens are indicated. These include young infants, especially with high white cell count and chromosomal abnormalities, or any patient with greater than $200 \times 10^9/l$ white cells at presentation. High-dose therapy with allogeneic bone marrow transplantation or autologous bone marrow rescue are under evaluation (Reaman et al., 1985; Sallan et al., 1989; Bordigoni et al., 1989; Schroeder, Pinkerton and Meller, 1991).

Relapses mostly occur within two years of stopping chemotherapy but children are generally not considered cured until they reach five years of continued remission and even then relapses beyond ten years may occur. Bone marrow relapse is the most common site, but extramedullary relapse in the central nervous system or the testis also occurs. The timing of relapse is of importance and disease recurring during continuing chemotherapy is unlikely to be curable, whereas relapse occurring years after cessation of treatment had a chance of salvage with alternative chemotherapy. This distinction is, however, less clear with intensive regimens using allogeneic marrow transplant (Brochstein *et al.*, 1987). One group of patients who do particularly well are those with an isolated testicular relapse occurring off treatment. After either orchidectomy or testicular irradiation and systemic reinduction chemotherapy, the majority of patients will remain in remission (Tiedemann, Chessells and Sandland, 1982). With isolated central nervous system relapse there is a high incidence of subsequent bone marrow relapse despite systemic retreatment (Pinkerton and Chessells, 1984). Repeat irradiation including the spine is necessary but total body irradiation with bone marrow transplant is an alternative.

Acute myeloid leukaemia

Lymphadenopathy is less common than in ALL and in the monocytic subgroup (M5) characteristic skin rashes or solid leukaemic deposits, e.g. orbital chloroma occur. Disseminated intravascular coagulation is associated with the promyelocytic hypergranular form (M3). This may occur at presentation or is a complication of initial chemotherapy due to release of granule content during blast lysis. The monocytic form may be associated with gingival, skin and CNS infiltration and often a very high white cell count. The diagnosis is made on morphological, cytochemical and surface marker characteristics.

The risk of CNS involvement is less than in ALL and intrathecal methotrexate alone is effective as CNS-directed treatment. Irradiation is rarely used. Other extramedullary manifestations such as testicular involvement are unusual (Chessells, O'Callaghan and Hardisty, 1986).

The drugs used in the induction of remission in AML are shown in Table 9.4 and with intensive induction regimens remission rates are over 80%. It seems unlikely that conventional continuing treatment as used in ALL is appropriate in AML and most regimens involve a short period of intensive pulsed or semi-continuous treatment. Patients who have HLA matched donors are generally treated in first remission, with high-dose therapy with allogeneic bone marrow transplantation. The role of high-dose procedures with autologous marrow rescue is currently under evaluation (Linch and Burnett, 1986).

Chronic leukaemias

Chronic granulocyte leukaemia (CGL) accounts for only 2–5% of all cases and chronic lymphocytic leukaemia is rarely, if ever, seen. CGL in childhood is generally divided into two types: the juvenile type and the adult type. The adult type presents in older children and is accompanied by marked splenomegaly, high white cell count and normal platelet count. Fetal haemoglobin level (HbF) is normal and the presence of Philadelphia chromosome t(9;22) in blast cells is pathognmonic. The juvenile type presents in younger children, usually under 4 years of age, is accompanied by splenomegaly and lymphadenopathy and often a characteristic lupus-like rash on the face. Presenting white cell count is usually lower than in the adult form, with a relative monocytosis and a high incidence of thrombocytopenia. HbF levels are usually raised to between 15 and 50%. The Philadelphia chromosome is not found. In addition to the differences in presenting features, the response to treatment also differs, the adult type shows a good response to busulphan, with a median survival of four years. By contrast, the juvenile type shows minimal response to chemotherapy and has a shorter median survival. The clinical course of Ph positive CGL is relatively indolent and treatment is aimed at controlling the white cell count using busulphan or hydroxyurea. Leucophoresis may be used as initial treatment where there is very high white cell count and the risk of hyperviscosity syndromes with cerebral infarction or priapism. Patients may remain in 'chronic phase' for months or years but eventually most will enter 'blast cell crisis'. These are heralded by bleeding, splenic enlargement and an increase in white cell count. There is usually myeloblastic transformation, although in a small percentage lymphoblastic leukaemia may develop. Treatment of the myeloblastic crisis is similar to that of AML. Allogeneic bone marrow transplantation during chronic phase offers the best chance of cure, with very low relapse rate following successful transplant (Gale and Champlin, 1986).

The juvenile type of CGL rarely shows a satisfactory response to conventional treatment or to high dose AML-type regimens. Patients usually die from infection or haemorrhage or may undergo blast transformation. Again, allogeneic transplantation holds the only hope for cure and this is best done without any attempt to achieve remission. Particularly intensive chemoradiotherapy preconditioning may be necessary to achieve graft take under these circumstances.

The monosomy 7 syndrome is a rare form of chronic myeloproliferative disease in children. The clinical presentation closely resembles juvenile CML, but without markedly raised HbF levels. The clonal abnormality of monosomy 7 in bone marrow is diagnostic (Sieff *et al.*, 1981).

9.2 LYMPHOMAS

Lymphomas are divided on the basis of histological features, immuno-phenotype history into two broad groups, Hodgkin's lymphoma and non-Hodgkin's lymphoma. Prognosis and treatment differ widely and therefore accurate initial diagnosis is essential.

Hodgkin's lymphoma

In Hodgkin's lymphoma/disease lymph nodes are infiltrated by a mixed cell population containing both the neoplastic component and a reactive inflammatory or stromal cell component. The origin of the Hodgkin's cell is unclear but it seems likely that it is of haemopoietic rather than connective tissue origin. The 'Rye' pathological classification is based upon both the predominant cell type and the microscopic structure (Kjeldsberg and Wilson, 1986). The commonest form in adolescence is the 'nodular sclerosing' form, characterized by bands of collagenous connective tissue encircling nodular areas of lymphoid tissue which contain an infiltrate of Hodgkin's cells. In the younger child the 'mixed cellularity' form predominates with diffuse cellular infiltrate of histiocytes, neutrophils, eosinophils, plasma cells and Hodgkin's cells. The 'lymphocyte predominant' group is composed almost entirely of lymphocytes and histiocytes with small clusters of Hodgkin's cells. This form is associated with a particularly good prognosis and it has been suggested that the heavy lymphocytic infiltration may reflect an immune response by the host. By contrast, the 'lymphocyte depleted' form, with predominant fibrosis and little reactive cellular infiltrate, has a poor prognosis. It should be emphasized that the prognostic importance of this pathological sub-classification has been reduced by the impact of effective chemotherapy.

There is a bimodal distribution with the first peak occurring at 15–30 years and the second at 45–55 years (Mueller, 1987). Less than 10% of all cases are in children under 15 and here the majority occur over 10 years of age. In Africa young children tend to be affected and often have mixed cellularity or lymphocyte depleted Hodgkin's disease. In the more socio-economically 'advanced' populations the age of onset is later and the more favourable histological types predominate. The disease is less common in children from large families or where there has been a high incidence of minor viral infections, suggesting that early exposure to the pathogen may reduce severity of subsequent illness. To date, however, no viral pathogen has been isolated in this disease, although the Epstein–Barr virus is an increasingly likely candidate (Jaffe, 1989).

Nodes in Hodgkin's disease are typically painless, rubbery and may have been present for several weeks, often varying in size. 80% present with disease on one or both sides of the neck and 60% have mediastinal disease (Figures 9.1, 9.2). Lymphadenopathy in the cervical and sub-mandibular regions frequently occurs with upper respiratory tract infections, but nodes in the lower neck and supraclavicular region are more suspicious. Associated symptoms reflecting systemic disease should be carefully sought, such as weight loss, night sweats and unexplained fever (so-called B symptoms), or persistent pruritus.

Initial investigations should include chest X-ray and ESR. Diagnosis rests on tissue biopsy, which should be of sufficient size to exclude reactive or infected nodes. Aspiration cytology is inadequate for the diagnosis of Hodgkin's disease. An accessible lymph node is usually possible to find, but occasionally with isolated mediastinal disease open biopsy is required. Staging investigations include CT scan of abdomen and thorax. Lymphangiography is no longer used in children, as the diagnostic yield over CT scan is minimal. As most patients now receive chemotherapy, precise delineation of nodes is of less importance. Similarly, staging splenectomy, although the most accurate way of defining involvement of the spleen, is no longer done. CT scan will provide adequate information and moreover isolated spleen involvement in the absence of nodal disease elsewhere is uncommon. In addition, there is operative morbidity with splenectomy and the risk of subsequent pneumococcal sepsis (Green *et al.*, 1983). Bone marrow trephine biopsy should be performed in patients with non-localized disease. Aspirate is inadequate due to patchy infiltration. The staging system of Ann Arbor is generally used (Table 9.5).

Treatment strategies differ between centres, with varying emphasis on the relative roles of radiotherapy and chemotherapy (Donaldson, 1984; Behrendt, van Bunningen and van Leeuwen, 1987; Selby, McElwain and

Table 9.5 Hodgkin's disease staging Ann Arbor classification

Clinical staging (CS)	
Pathological staging (laparotomy) is *not* done in children	
Stage I	Involvement of a single lymph node region (I) or of a single extralymphatic organ or site (I_E)
Stage II	Involvement of two or more lymph node regions on the same side of the diaphragm (II) or localized involvement of extralymphatic organ or site and of 1 or more lymph node regions on the same side of the diaphragm (II_E)
Stage III	Involvement of lymph node regions on both sides of the diaphragm (III) which may also be accompanied by localized involvement of extralymphatic organ or site (III_E) or by involvement of the spleen (III_S) or both (III_{SE})
Stage IV	Disseminated involvement of one or more extralymphatic organs or tissues with or without associated lymph node involvement

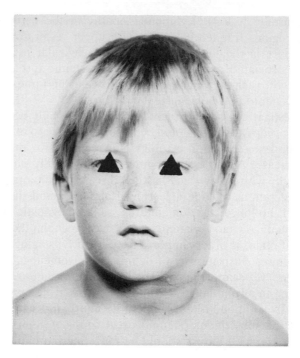

Figure 9.1 Lymphadenopathy in the left cervical and supraclavicular region in a boy with Hodgkin's disease.

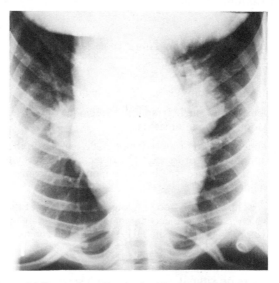

Figure 9.2 Bilateral hilar and mediastinal widening in Hodgkin's disease.

Canellos, 1987). Although high cure rates are achieved with extended field irradiation, even in stage III patients, the sequelae in growing children is unacceptable and the trend is therefore towards chemotherapy alone for most patients. In the current UKCCSG regimen, involved field irradiation (30 Gy) is given only to stage I patients. Bilateral fields are used to reduce neck asymmetry (Figure 9.1). With this approach, up to one-fifth of patients with stage I disease will relapse but the majority, if not all, are curable with subsequent chemotherapy. All other stages receive chemotherapy (ChlVPP). With regimens such as ChlVPP (chlorambucil, vinblastine, procarbazine, prednisolone), MOPP (mustine, vincristine, procarbazine, prednisolone) or ABVD (adriamycin, bleomycin, vincristine, DTIC) 6–8 courses usually are given (Table 9.6) (Jenkin *et al.*, 1982; Robinson *et al.*, 1984). Concern about the sterilizing effect and the small but significant risk of second malignancies associated with the use of multiple alkylating agent chemotherapy, has led to interest in new combinations containing drugs such as etoposide. If these are shown to be equally effective then there is an argument for extending chemotherapy alone to include stage I patients.

Additional irradiation is often given to patients with initially bulky mediastinal disease, greater than one-third the transthoracic diameter. Here the radiation generally includes the neck and axillary nodal group (Figure 9.2). Recent studies suggest that radiotherapy may not be necessary, even in these patients, provided a complete response is achieved with chemotherapy (Ekert *et al.*, 1988). A small residual mediastinal mass may be fibrosis and gallium scan or biopsy should be used to decide whether irradiation is necessary (Weiner, Leventhal and Cantor, 1991).

Late relapses may occur in Hodgkin's disease and therefore prolonged follow-up is required before one can say that the patient is cured (Russell *et al.*, 1984).

Non-Hodgkin's lymphoma (NHL)

This malignant proliferation of lymphoid precursor cells has a similar cellular origin to leukaemia and shares many of the immunohistochemical

Table 9.6 Treatment strategy in Hodgkin's disease

Stage I	Local involved field irradiation ~30 Gy
Stage II–IV	ChlVPP chemotherapy × 6–8 courses depending on speed of response
	Irradiation only biopsy-proven residual disease

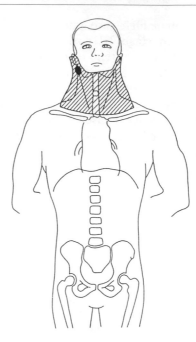

Figure 9.3 Limited field, excluding the clavicles, for a single cervical node.

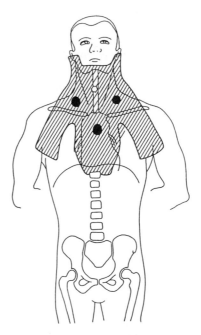

Figure 9.4 Limited involved field with mediastinal involvement.

and biological markers. Lymph nodes are the predominant site of disease with, in some cases, secondary involvement of the bone marrow, central nervous system and other organs. Local irradiation was in the past curative in a small number of cases but with the advent of effective chemotherapy this now has little role.

Complex classifications of lymphomas are found in adult oncology, devised on the basis of histological features and natural history. Low-grade tumours, often nodular or follicular, behave in a comparatively benign manner, whereas high-grade or diffuse tumours are more aggressive. In children, low-grade tumours almost never occur and a much simpler classification has been evolved to subdivide the high-grade tumours on the basis of morphology and immune markers. There are four main categories: diffuse lymphoblastic, T cell or B cell, lymphoblastic non-B non-T and 'others' (Table 9.7). The last group includes rare subtypes, such as the large cell anaplastic lymphoma, distinguished by positivity for K1 antigen (CD30). This disease covers a spectrum of clinical presentations from localized skin disease to disseminated tumour. Peripheral T-cell lymphoma contains relatively mature T cells. Malignant histiocytosis is a rare disseminated disease presenting with weight loss and fever.

The presentation of NHL depends on the site of initial disease. There may be extensive cervical lymphadenopathy. T-cell NHL can present with rapidly progressive upper airway obstruction and superior vena caval obstruction (Figure 9.5). B cell NHL in the abdomen presents with pain

Table 9.7 NHL classification

Lymphoblastic B cell	Surface Ig (+) B marker (+) e.g. CD19 TdT (−) FAB L3 marrow or CSF Ig gene rearrangement t(8;14), t(8;22), t(3;8)
Lymphoblastic T cell	TdT (+), acid phosphatase (+) T marker (+) e.g. CD 2–4 FAB L1 or L2 marrow or CSF T cell receptor gene rearrangement
Lymphoblastic non-B/non-T	CALLA positive, including pre-B cell: cytoplasmic μ (+)
Large cell anaplastic	Ki-1 (+) (CD30)
Peripheral T cell lymphoma including pleomorphic T cell	
True histiocytic and malignant histiocytosis	

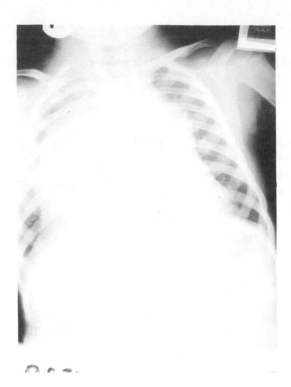

Figure 9.5 Marked anterior mediastinal widening in a boy with T-lymphoblastic lymphoma who presented with respiratory distress.

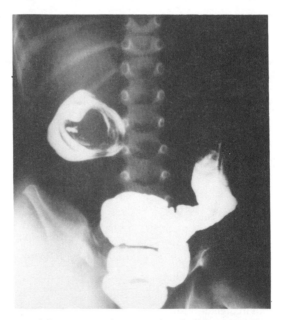

Figure 9.6 Ileocaecal intussusception associated with a nodal mass in abdominal non-Hodgkin's lymphoma.

or a palpable mass. Involvement in the ileum may cause intussusception (Figure 9.6). With advanced disease there may be ascites and marked weight loss. Liver, spleen and kidney infiltration also may occur. Marrow and CSF involvement occur in both T and B NHL. Patients with greater than 25% infiltration of bone marrow are classified as 'leukaemia' and in the case of B-cell disease this form is associated with a particularly high incidence of CNS and testicular disease. Those with less than 25% marrow infiltration are classified as stage IV disease.

African Burkitt's lymphoma (endemic Burkitt's), shares a common cellular origin but is a separate clinical entity from European 'Burkitt's disease'. It typically affects males between 6 and 8 years and involves the jaw, abdomen and CNS. The association with EB virus is clear (Chapter 2).

Routine staging investigations in NHL define the extent of nodal involvement with chest X-ray and abdominal ultrasound or CT body scan. As chemotherapy is given to all patients, precise definition of nodal involvement is less important than in Hodgkin's disease and CT scan is not an absolute prerequisite. Bone marrow aspirate and spinal fluid cytology are examined. Bone marrow trephine biopsy may be done but tumour infiltration is usually diffuse and seen on an aspirate. The most commonly used staging system is that devised by Murphy (Table 9.8).

Irradiation of nodal disease plays no useful role in the treatment of T or B NHL. Urgent cyto-reduction in the case of tracheal compression can be achieved as rapidly with chemotherapy as with radiotherapy. Irradiation of initial bulk nodal disease following chemotherapy has no value. In

Table 9.8 Murphy classification for childhood NHL

I	A single tumour (extranodal) or single anatomical area (nodal) with the exclusion of the mediastinum or abdomen.
II	A single tumour (extranodal) with regional node involvement. Two or more nodal areas on the same side of the diaphragm. Two single (extranodal) tumours with or without regional node involvement of the same side of the diaphragm. A primary gastrointestinal tract tumour, usually in the ileocaecal area, with or without involvement of associated mesenteric nodes only, grossly completely resected.
III	Two single tumours (extranodal) on opposite sides of the diaphragm. Two or more nodal areas above and below the diaphragm. *All* primary intrathoracic tumours (mediastinal, pleural, thymic). *All* extensive primary intra-abdominal disease, unresected. *All* paraspinal or epidural tumours, regardless of other tumour site(s).
IV	Any of the above with initial CNS and/or bone marrow involvement.

some studies cranial irradiation is used in T-cell disease for CNS directed therapy, but as in B NHL intrathecal chemotherapy and high-dose systemic methotrexate is probably sufficient, unless there is CNS involvement at presentation.

Surgery should only be used to obtain a tissue diagnosis, although marrow, ascitic fluid or pleural effusion cytology often provide the diagnosis. There is no role for initial debulking of abdominal disease and any attempt at resection of either abdominal or thoracic NHL causes unnecessary morbidity without therapeutic benefit.

It has been clearly shown that chemotherapy for NHL should be selected on the basis of histological and immune sub-type. T-cell disease is best treated in the same way as T-cell leukaemia, with multi-agent induction, consolidation and two years' continuing treatment (Wheeler and Chessells, 1990). Five-year survival is similar to ALL, ~60%. B-cell NHL is best treated with a short pulsed regimen usually based on cyclophosphamide and methotrexate with a duration of between six and nine months. With this approach survival rates are high, stage I and II 95%, III 80% and IV 60%. With localized B-cell disease it may be possible to devise non-sterilizing, non-alkylating agent regimens (Table 9.9). For advanced B-cell disease with multi-organ involvement or CNS disease the cure rate in the past has been extremely poor. The introduction of very intensive regimens including high-dose cyclophosphamide, cytarabine and methotrexate and intensive intrathecal therapy have produced a striking improvement in this small group of patients (Patte *et al.*, 1986; Philip *et al.*, 1987). This approach is, however, associated inevitably with a high treatment-related morbidity.

9.3 BRAIN TUMOURS

Intracranial neoplasms are the commonest solid tumours in childhood. There are several histological sub-groups (Tables 9.10, 9.11). In children the commonest tumours are low-grade astrocytoma and medulloblastoma.

Table 9.9 Treatment strategy in non-Hodgkin's lymphoma

Localized: Stages I and II
6 months of low morbidity chemotherapy, e.g. cyclophosphamide, vincristine, doxorubicin, prednisone ± methotrexate, cytarabine, thioguanine
Intrathecal methotrexate only to head and neck primaries

Non-localized: Stages II and IV
6 months of the same drugs but at higher doses and high dose intensity.
Add CNS directed therapy such as high dose cytarabine for high risk B ALL or CNS positive or refractory disease

---

Table 9.10 Histological classification of brain tumours

Gliomas
   Astrocytoma
   Ependymoma
   Oligodendroglioma
   Glioblastoma
   Mixed glioma
Neuroectodermal tumours
   Medulloblastoma
   PNET (primitive neuroectodermal tumour)
Neurinoma
   Optic nerve glioma
Pineal
   Pineoblastoma
   Pineocytoma
Germ cell
   Germinoma
   Teratoma – differentiated
               undifferentiated
Craniopharyngioma

Table 9.11 Classification of brain tumours based on primary site

Supratentorial		Cerebral astrocytoma
		frontal
		temporal
		parietal
		Lateral ventricle ependymoma
		Craniopharyngioma
	Especially <1 year {	Primitive neuroectodermal tumour
		Choroid plexus papilloma
		Meningioma
		Teratoma
Infratentorial		Astrocytoma
		Medulloblastoma
		Brain stem glioma
		3rd ventricle ependymoma
Intraspinal	Extradural	Neuroblastoma
		Sarcoma
		Lymphoma
	Intradural	Neurofibromatosis
		Dermoid
		Lipomata
	Intramedullary	Astrocytoma

Lesions such as neuroma, meningioma and pituitary tumours are less frequently seen in children than in adults. Tumour sub-types and their usual location are listed in Table 9.11.

Diagnosis

Symptoms are related to either raised intracranial pressure or a mass effect due to a space occupying lesion. Severe recurrent or persisting headaches are relatively rare in children and these should be viewed with a high index of suspicion. Early morning vomiting and nausea or subtle alterations in behaviour occur. In small infants there may be rapid or slowly progressive development of macrocephaly with prominent bulging anterior fontanelle. With the more indolent low-grade gliomas a large head or wide fontanelle may be detected at routine checks. Focal third or sixth cranial nerve palsies may occur.

The signs due to a space occupying lesion depend on the site. Medulloblastoma will often produce cerebellar ataxia and nystagmus; parietal tumours, focal weakness; supra-chiasmal lesions, visual disturbance with nystagmus; brain stem lesions; extensive cranial nerve palsies.

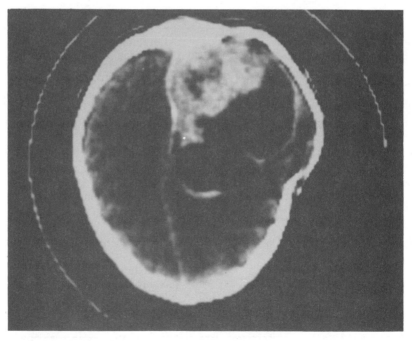

Figure 9.7 CT scan of large cystic primitive neuroectodermal tumour involving the cerebral hemisphere.

Clinical examination may localize the lesion but the mainstay of diagnostic studies is the CT scan (Figure 9.7). This has replaced invasive procedures such as cerebral arterial angiography or air ventriculography. For children under 4 years old a general anaesthetic or heavy sedation is usually necessary for satisfactory imaging. The use of intravenous contrast is essential and may aid both detection of small lesions and delineation of the tumour extent. Magnetic resonance imaging (MRI) has an advantage over CT scan with regard to the clarity of anatomical detail (Figure 9.8) and is superior to CT scan for imaging brain stem lesions and some posterior fossa lesions. It is also an invaluable tool for evaluation of spinal masses.

Surgery plays an important role in initial management. Insertion of a ventriculo-peritoneal or ventriculo-atrial shunt may produce improved symptoms by relieving raised intracranial pressure. Wherever possible, complete resection should be performed and in the extent of initial surgery remains a major factor in the likelihood of cure. If complete

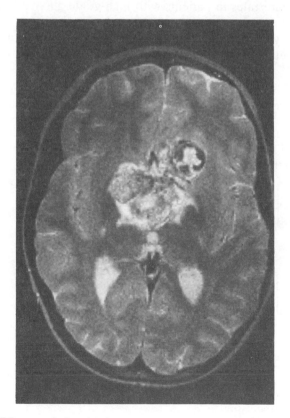

Figure 9.8 MRI scan of pineal teratoma.

resection is impossible, debulking may have a role in relieving local compression. An important function of surgery is to provide tissue for histological diagnosis. In the past, radiotherapy has been standard treatment for the majority of lesions irrespective of histology and therefore the pathological sub-type was not of major importance. With attempts to refine radiotherapy techniques and the development of new chemotherapy strategies, it is important that histology is obtained in patients if at all possible. In small children with deep inaccessible tumours, e.g. thalamic, pineal, mid-brain or brainstem, this is often difficult but stereotactic techniques may be useful. Under general anaesthesia the skull is fixed in position and the biopsy needle directed towards a predetermined site based on computerized CT or MRI imaging. Using this approach the majority of patients can be biopsied with low morbidity (Thomas, Anderson and du Boulay, 1984; Thomas *et al.*, 1986).

Radiotherapy is usually given after surgery and doses of between 40 and 50 Gy to the primary site are given, fractionated over several weeks. With inoperable lesions this may be the sole therapy. Because of the disappointing cure rates in patients with high-grade gliomas and inoperable medulloblastomas, there is increasing interest in the use of chemotherapy to improve cytotoxic effect and there is also major concern about neurological sequelae in small infants; moreover, irradiation of the spinal axis

Table 9.12 Treatment strategies following surgery in brain tumours

Radiotherapy only   – high grade glioma
                    – ependymoma

Combination therapy – medulloblastoma; PNET

| Carboplatin Vincristine Etoposide | alternating with | Cyclophosphamide Etoposide Vincristine | → IRRAD |

Chemotherapy alone – infant PNET

| Carboplatin Vincristine Etoposide | high dose methotrexate | Cyclophosphamide Etoposide Vincristine | × 12/12 |

                    – optic glioma

Vincristine/actinomycin

        or   × 12/12

Vincristine/carboplatin

produces significant vertebral growth retardation (Shalet *et al.*, 1987). In some tumours whole brain doses of up to 35 Gy are electively used. If effective chemotherapy could be found radiation doses could be reduced or in selected cases even omitted (Table 9.12).

Tumour subtypes

Astrocytomas are divided into two broad groups – low grade (I and II) and high grade (III and IV) depending on histological features. Low-grade tumours (e.g. pilocytic and fibrillary astrocytomas) tend to be pleomorphic with cells containing oval nuclei and dense chromation aggregates. There may be stellate structures, giant cells and microcystic formation. Epithelial proliferation may be seen and mitotic activity is generally low. By contrast, the high-grade tumours (e.g. anaplastic astrocytoma and glioblastoma multiforme) contain many mitotic figures and polymorphic nuclei with high nuclear cytoplasmic ratio. The lesions may be necrotic and highly vascularized (Russell and Rubinstein, 1977). Overall cure rate for low-grade gliomas (Grades I and II) is around 60% at 5 years and for high grade 25% (Bloom, 1982; Woo, Donaldson and Cox, 1988). Chemotherapy combinations including such agents as vincristine, actinomycin, CCNU and cisplatin have to date had little impact on survival with either low- or high-grade gliomas, although responses have been intensely reported (Pendergrass *et al.*, 1987). One American randomized study has, however, demonstrated significant benefit with adjuvant vincristine, CCNU and prednisolone (Sposto *et al.*, 1989). Some tumours may behave in a very indolent manner and in a small child if symptoms are minimal or have resolved with a shunt procedure a 'wait and watch' policy, with regular review CT scans, may be justified. Definitive irradiation is withheld unless there is evidence of disease progression (Allen *et al.*, 1986).

Ependymomas make up about 10% of brain tumours and arise from the lining of the ventricles. They occur with equal frequency above and below the tentorium and tend to be differentiated, well circumscribed lesions, suggestive of a benign character. They may, however, behave in an aggressive manner, extending laterally into the cerebellar pontine angle or inferiorly through the foramen magnum and down the cervical cord. There is also a tendency to seed into the spinal fluid and for this reason whole neuraxis radiotherapy is recommended for high-grade ependymomas and all posterior fossa lesions of any grade. A dose of 50 Gy to the primary tumour and 30 Gy to the neuraxis is standard practice. Survival at 10 years follow-up is around 40% but tends to be lower for supratentorial primaries (Bloom, 1982). No benefit from chemotherapy has been reported to date.

Medulloblastoma is the commonest infratentorial tumour. The tumour is composed of small uniform cells with hyperchromatic, angular or carrot-shaped nuclei. There is high mitotic activity and often focal necrosis and vascular proliferation. Tumours contain variable degrees of neuronal differentiation with rosette formation or astrocytic differentiation. The desmoplastic sub-group contains strands of connective tissue with nests of malignant cells. This type tends to be superficial and resectable, thus carrying a good prognosis. The commonest site for medulloblastoma is in the midline of the cerebellum and the tumour tends to seed early to CSF (Figure 9.9). Rarely, extracerebral metastases to bone and bone marrow occur. Boys are affected twice as commonly as girls and tend to have a worse prognosis. The initial work up should include myelography and CSF cytology, as intraspinal deposits may necessitate higher local doses of radiation. Medulloblastoma is the brain tumour in which chemotherapy has been most extensively evaluated. The European SIOP group and the American CCSG have carried out randomized prospective studies of the value of combinations of vincristine, CCNU and steroids and have shown a significant benefit for younger patients and those with incomplete resection or brain stem involvement (Allen *et al.*, 1986). More recently, regimens have been designed to give chemotherapy, 'sandwiched' between surgery and radiotherapy. Reduced doses of irradiation to the whole brain and spinal column in selected sub-groups of patients are also under evaluation as are new drug combinations, including cisplatin, etoposide

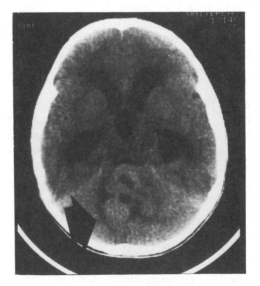

Figure 9.9 CT scan image of cerebellar medulloblastoma.

and ifosfamide. Current 5-year survival is around 50% and bad prognostic features include age less than 5 years, male sex, incomplete resection, involvement of brain stem or vermis, and non-desmoplastic pathology (Silverman *et al.*, 1984; Pendergrass *et al.*, 1987; Walker and Allen, 1988).

Primitive neuroectodermal tumour (PNET) is the supratentorial counterpart of the medulloblastoma. It is highly malignant with a tendency to spread to the cerebrospinal fluid and occasionally to extracerebral sites. This tumour is of particular interest as it is chemosensitive and occurs in the younger child where irradiation should be avoided if possible. There is an increasing trend to group medulloblastoma and cerebral PNET as a single tumour, i.e. cranial PNET as the two are probably biologically identical.

The cerebellar astrocytoma is a more indolent tumour with two histological sub-types; the juvenile piloid tumour with elongated unipolar cells and fibrillary structure, or the diffuse less differentiated variety. The tumours may be cystic or multicystic and, where resectable, there is a 90% chance of cure.

Brain stem gliomas tend to present early due to their anatomical localization in a region of densely packed neurological pathways (Figure 9.10). Most tumours arise in the pons and are of low-grade histology but despite

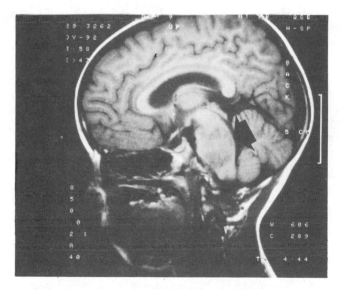

Figure 9.10 Magnetic resonance image of brain stem glioma.

this are particularly difficult to treat. Radiotherapy remains the mainstay of treatment but cure rates are generally less than 20%. Because of the site, biopsy is frequently difficult and the differential diagnosis rests between a simple cyst, granuloma and focal encephalitis and without stereotactic biopsy a small number of benign lesions will be irradiated. Because of the poor outlook with radiotherapy this group is under study with more aggressive chemotherapy (Johnson *et al.*, 1987; Wolff, Phillips and Herzig, 1987).

Optic gliomas are low-grade astrocytomas presenting with a mass at the optic chiasma or along the optic nerve (Figure 9.11). About 25% are associated with von Recklinghausen's syndrome. The tumour may extend to the pituitary fossa producing hypopituitarism, to the hypothalamus producing precocious puberty or secondary hypopituitarism, or obstruct the foramen of Munro leading to hydrocephalus. Differential diagnosis of a chiasmal mass includes craniopharyngioma, meningioma, suprasellar germinoma, hypothalamic glioma and dermoid cyst. Biopsy is usually

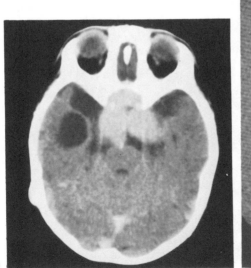
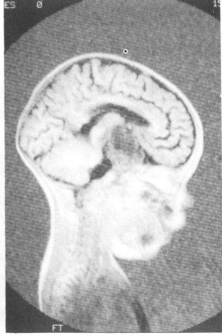

(a)

Figure 9.11 (a) CT scan and (b) magnetic resonance image of infant with glioma involving the optic nerve tract.

possible in these tumours but decisions regarding therapy may be difficult. Being histologically low grade, growth may be very slow. Symptom progression can be minimal and obstructive hydrocephalus will improve with shunting. In unilateral cases tumour resection may be possible but evidence that radiotherapy is necessary in all cases is lacking. Radiation is usually recommended for older children and the overall outcome is good, with survival over 70% (Horwich and Bloom, 1985). In the small infant a 'wait and watch' policy may be applied as in the case of other low-grade astrocytomas. Recent reports suggest that low-dose, frequent administration, chemotherapy with vincristine and actinomycin or carboplatin may have useful activity in these tumours (Packer et al., 1988).

Pineal tumours include the true pineoblastoma, an embryonal tumour of pineal tissue. This is a highly malignant tumour which is usually radiosensitive. Suprasellar germinomas are malignant germ cell tumours arising at an abnormal site on the migration pathway of germ cells during embryonal development. These may be associated with elevated levels of alpha-fetoprotein in the CSF and are highly radio- and chemosensitive. Cure rate should be high and in the small child chemotherapy alone may be curative (Allen, Kim and Packer, 1987).

Craniopharyngiomas are slow growing histologically benign tumours which are often cystic. Excision is usually difficult and complete resection is rare. In general, non-radical surgery minimizing normal tissue damage is recommended. Aspiration alone may be appropriate followed by irradiation and cure rates in the region of 80% are to be expected (Mananka, Teramoto and Takakura, 1985).

Meningiomas are rarely seen in young children but may affect male adolescents. These are usually supratentorial, and occur in the cerebral hemisphere convexities, the parasagittal falx, the lateral ventricle, the orbit and the sphenoid petrous ridge. Multiple meningiomas occur in von Recklinghausen's disease. Because of their situation these tumours are usually resectable and no radiation is required.

Intraspinal tumours are also uncommon (Table 9.11). The presenting symptoms depend on the level involved and the rapidity of tumour growth. Motor weakness with limp or abnormality of gait are seen and back or root pain may occur. Sacral lesions may lead to bladder or bowel dysfunction. With very slow growing lesions musculoskeletal abnormalities may develop. Investigation should include plain X-ray, CT scan and MRI. The last may be of particular use in defining the anatomical distribution. Myelography is still recommended by some but is not without hazard and may exacerbate symptoms.

Occasionally treatment is with chemotherapy alone, as in the cases of lymphoma or neuroblastoma, where the diagnosis may be made without biopsy. More often initial surgery is indicated and resection may be possible, perhaps using ultrasonic aspiration technique. The use of radiotherapy or adjuvant chemotherapy depends on the tumour type.

9.4 NEUROBLASTOMA

Fetal neural cells (neuroblasts) migrate from the neural crest to the sympathetic ganglia and adrenal gland. Neuroblastoma may arise at any site where sympathetic neural tissue is normally found (Figure 9.12).

This is the commonest intra-abdominal tumour in children and the median age of presentation is 2 years. It is occasionally seen in adolescents or even adults. Primitive neuroblastic tissue resembling tumour is found in 0.5–2% of autopsies of children under 3 months old, suggesting a high rate of spontaneous regression of 'neuroblastoma *in situ*'.

Approximately 40% arise in the adrenal, 40% in other abdominal sites and 15% in the thorax. Rarely, ectopic forms arise in the kidney. Associated abnormalities include cardiac and genito-urinary anomalies, neurofibromatosis, Hirschsprung's disease and heterochromia iridis.

The aetiology of neuroblastoma is unknown, but it seems likely that there are at least two distinct biological entities, ranging from stage 4S which spontaneously regresses, resembling 'neuroblastoma *in situ*', to the highly aggressive metastatic form presenting at over 1 year of age. Correlations between a number of biological characteristics and advanced stage disease provide tantalizing clues to the mechanism of malignant behaviour but little about the primary defect. Amplification of the proto-oncogene myc-n, deletions on chromosome 1 and a nuclear DNA content (ploidy) close to normal (i.e. diploid) all carry a poor prognosis (Look *et al.*, 1991).

Neuroblastoma most commonly presents as an abdominal mass with systemic features due to metastatic disease including weight loss, general malaise, bone and joint pain, anaemia and fever. Hypertension is due either to catecholamine release or renal vascular compression and diarrhoea has been reported due to the release of vasoactive intestinal peptides by tumour. Focal neurological signs may be present if there is primary intraspinal disease, extension of paravertebral disease into the spinal cord, or if there is compression of pelvic nerves. Intracranial metastases occur but are very rare. A specific sub-group presenting with cerebellar ataxia and usually associated with a well-differentiated intra-thoracic primary has a particularly good prognosis. The mechanism for the cerebellar toxicity, which may either precede the development of

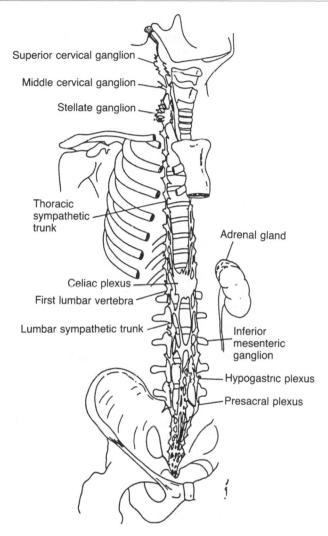

Figure 9.12 Sites where sympathetic nerve tissue is found which may be the site of primary disease in neuroblastoma. 40% arise in the adrenal, 40% at other abdominal sites and 15% in the thorax.

demonstrable tumour or occur after resection of the primary tumour, is unknown. It has been suggested that it may be immunological due to autoantibody cross-reactivity between neuroblastoma and cerebral neural tissue. The associated nystagmus has led to the term 'dancing eyes syndrome'.

There is not infrequently a long history of persistent or recurrent abdominal pain ascribed to other causes, such as 'growing pains', epiphysitis, arthritis – septic or rheumatoid, until the systemic features develop. Subtle radiological abnormalities may be missed and the child with pelvic or femoral pain treated for 'irritable hip' before a diagnosis is reached. Exophthalmos and peri-orbital discoloration due to disease infiltration may occur. Thoracic tumours may be detected at the time of chest X-ray for another cause.

The diagnostic criteria defined by the International Neuroblastoma Study Group are a biopsy sample diagnosis or unequivocal marrow infiltrate plus raised catecholamines (Brodeur et al., 1988). The prerequisite of a tissue diagnosis if marrow is involved is debatable and elevated urinary catecholamines with a suprarenal mass on CT scan is often considered diagnostic. There is, however, an increasing trend towards biopsy of all primary tumours in order to obtain information regarding the histological sub-type, myc-n amplification, tumour karyotype and ploidy, all of which may predict the aggressiveness of the disease. The urine metabolites, homovanillic acid (HVA) and vanillyl mandelic acid (VMA), are raised in about 85% of patients and dopamine is raised in about 90% of patients. In the past, 24-hour urine collections have been recommended in order to avoid false negative results due to the episodic nature of catecholaminic release from the tumour. The sensitivity of assays is now improved and a random sample in which the catecholamine metabolites are quantitated in relation to the creatinine content is adequate. Around 10% of patients are metabolite negative. There is no correlation between the degree of elevation of urinary metabolites, although a disproportionately high HVA:VMA content indicates a less differentiated tumour and a poorer prognosis (Evans et al., 1987).

Skeletal surveys are now rarely used as technetium bone scan is more accurate. With increasing experience of mIBG scanning this technique may supersede the bone scan, because it is more sensitive and also being disease specific it resolves rapidly with response, unlike the technetium scan (Figure 9.13). However, it may be difficult to distinguish patchy bone marrow disease from bone lesions and if the latter proves to be of prognostic value then technetium scan may remain an important staging investigation. MRI can also be used to demonstrate marrow disease (Figure 9.14). Because of the patchy nature of bone marrow involvement in neuroblastoma, a single aspirate is totally inadequate for documenting marrow metastases. Trephine biopsies are essential. Immunological studies using antibodies against neuroblastoma cells may further improve sensitivity (Moss et al., 1991).

Pathological sub-groups have been devised in an attempt to assess prognosis more accurately. Most, such as that of Shimada, are based on the degree of differentiation, ranging from the highly differentiated,

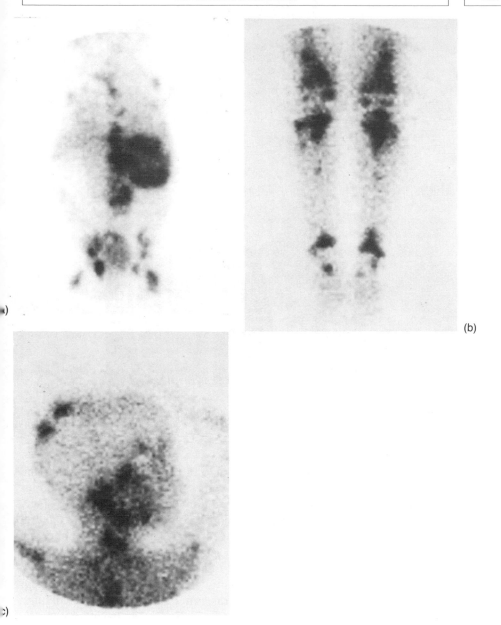

(b)

Figure 9.13 ^{123}I mIBG scans demonstrating uptake in the abdomen and multiple bone and bone marrow sites (a), uptake around the knees and ankles (b) and in the skull (c). Uptake is normally seen in the parotid region and salivary glands, also in the thyroid if inadequately blocked with potassium iodide prior to the scan.

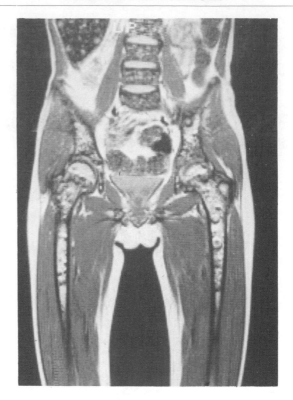

Figure 9.14 Magnetic resonance image showing extensive low signal in the femora indicating tumour infiltration.

relatively benign, ganglioneuroblastoma to the highly undifferentiated and malignant small round cell neuroblastoma. In the differentiated tumour there is a high percentage of mature ganglion cells dispersed either singly or in groups through a background matrix composed of primitive neural tissue with Schwannian sheaths and myelination, and a fibrous supporting framework. The less differentiated ganglioneuroblastoma contains a mixture of differentiated and undifferentiated sympathetoblasts, often arranged in rosettes. The undifferentiated form may have few clear diagnostic features to distinguish it from other small round cell tumours; supportive evidence may then be obtained from electron microscopical demonstration of neurosecretory granules and cytoplasmic neuronal processes. Immunological markers using monoclonal antibodies raised against fetal brain tissue react semi-specifically with neuroblastoma and a panel of such markers may be helpful in making a diagnosis (Kemshead & Pritchard, 1984).

The likelihood of cure depends on the stage of disease and age.

Table 9.13 INSS staging system for neuroblastoma

Stage 1	Localized tumour confined to the area of origin; complete gross excision, with or without microscopic residual disease; identifiable ipsilateral and contralateral lymph nodes negative microscopically
Stage 2A	Unilateral tumour with incomplete gross excision; identifiable ipsilateral and contralateral lymph nodes negative microscopically
Stage 2B	Unilateral tumour with complete or incomplete gross excision; with positive ipsilateral regional lymph nodes; identifiable contralateral lymph nodes negative microscopically
Stage 3	Tumour infiltrating across the midline with or without regional lymph node involvement; or, unilateral tumour with contralateral regional lymph node involvement; or, midline tumour with bilateral regional lymph node involvement
Stage 4	Dissemination of tumour to distant lymph nodes, bone, bone marrow, liver and/or other organs (except as defined in stage 4S)
Stage 4S	Localized primary tumour as defined for stage 1 or 2 with dissemination limited to liver, skin and/or bone marrow

Table 9.14 Treatment strategy in neuroblastoma

Stages 1 & 2A	Surgery alone
2B	OPEC/OJEC × 6 courses then surgery
3	OPEC/OJEC × 6–8 courses then surgery; irradiation if incomplete resection
4	OPEC/OJEC or more intensive high dose intensity variant then surgery; *high dose melphalan with autologous marrow rescue
4S	Observe; low dose irradiation or chemotherapy if required
OPEC/OJEC	Vincristine, cisplatin or carboplatin (JM8) alternately, etoposide, cyclophosphamide

*Not given to infants <1 year at diagnosis

Additional prognostic factors include the serum neurone-specific enolase, LDH, serum ferritin (Evans *et al.*, 1987) and the biological features described earlier.

The INSS staging system is shown in Table 9.13 (Brodeur *et al.*, 1988). Stage 1 and 2 tumours are usually well differentiated with few adverse prognostic features and are curable by surgery alone. It is likely that some such tumours remain quiescent and may even resolve spontaneously. The decision to remove an asymptomatic thoracic ganglioneuroma is based

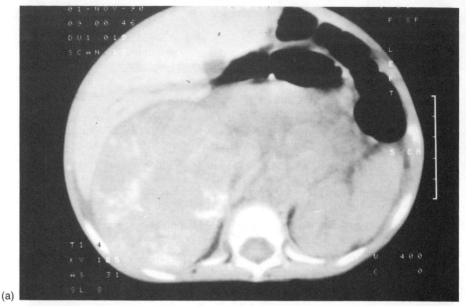

(a)

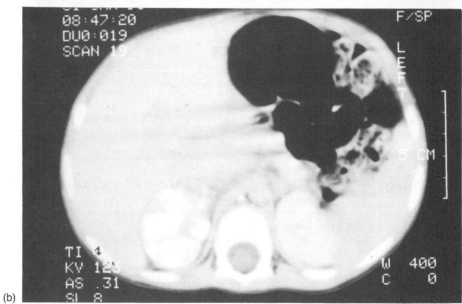

(b)

Figure 9.15 A calcified right suprarenal neuroblastoma before therapy (a), following treatment the mass typically shrinks with increased calcification (b).

more on grounds of allaying anxiety than clear evidence that such a tumour will progress or metastasize. There is evidence that microscopic residue after resection of such lesions does not lead to recurrence in the majority of patients (Matthay *et al.*, 1989). Neither radiation nor chemotherapy is necessary for localized disease unless there is nodal involvement (stage 2B) when a short course of chemotherapy should be given (Table 9.14). Stage 3 disease is unresectable at presentation, but preoperative chemotherapy will usually shrink the mass sufficiently to permit complete resection (Figure 9.15). Improvements in the efficacy of chemotherapy and in surgical technique have led to improved survival in such patients which should exceed 60% at 5 years. Stage 4 disease with metastases to bone marrow, bone, liver, nodes or skin has been regarded as incurable. There is, however, increasing evidence that with intensive chemotherapy between 10 and 20% of such patients will survive (Pritchard *et al.*, 1987). The site of metastatic disease influences prognosis, being better for those with distant nodal involvement alone and worst for those with multiple bony metastases. Age is the strongest prognostic feature and patients under 18 months do significantly better than older children.

Management of stage 4 neuroblastoma involves a combination of chemotherapy, surgery and radiotherapy. Current chemotherapy regimens include cisplatin and the epidophyllotoxins VM26 or etoposide in combination with vincristine and cyclophosphamide or ifosfamide. In about two-thirds of patients there will be complete clearance of metastatic disease and surgical resection of the primary is usually recommended. Complete resection or resection with only microscopic residue is achieved in about half the patients. As in stage 3 tumours, local irradiation either as external beam or mIBG targetted irradiation may have a role in treating residual disease (Lewis *et al.*, 1991). The use of high-dose chemoradiotherapy for patients in first remission is currently under evaluation but a randomized study using high-dose melphalan with autologous marrow rescue in responding patients produced a significant prolongation of progression free survival (Pritchard *et al.*, 1986). The value of multiagent regimens, often containing total body irradiation, has yet to be proved (Philip *et al.*, 1987; Shuster *et al.*, 1991).

Stage 4S neuroblastoma

This occurs almost only in infants under 1 year of age. Despite extensive infiltration of bone marrow, liver and skin, the disease will usually resolve spontaneously over several months. The primary site is generally suprarenal and of small volume. The features which distinguish stage 4S from stage 4 in young infants are the presence of bony metastases or distant nodal metastases. The latter are true stage 4 and require intensive chemotherapy but their outlook is comparatively good (Kretschmar *et al.*, 1984).

Although stage 4S is self-limiting, early morbidity does occur. This is often due to the massive hepatomegaly with splinting of the diaphragm and consequent respiratory distress (Figure 9.16). The resultant mortality may be as high as 15–20%, from respiratory insufficiency combined with sepsis or complications of treatment (Wilson *et al.*, 1991). An initial 'wait and watch' policy is appropriate but at the first sign of significant respiratory embarrassment low-dose radiation (4–8 Gy) should be given to the liver, or small doses of chemotherapy, e.g. vincristine or low-dose cyclophosphamide (Suarez *et al.*, 1991). This usually produces tumour shrinkage and resolution of symptoms. In the past, surgical procedures such as insertion of a silastic bag to allow expansion of abdominal contents has been used, but this is now rarely performed. Progression to true stage 4 disease occurs in less than 10% of patients and may be predictable by study of biological features (Bourhis *et al.*, 1989).

Screening

Measuring urine catecholamine metabolites at six months has been suggested as a method of population 'screening' for neuroblastoma. Preliminary studies in Japan have indicated that this may reduce the number that progress to metastatic disease. It seems likely, however, that with this approach a number of innocent 'tumours' which would have resolved spontaneously will be treated. The method is currently under evaluation in the UK, France and USA (Murphy *et al.*, 1991).

9.5 WILMS' TUMOUR

Wilms' tumour or nephroblastoma is an embryonal cancer arising in the metanephric blastema cell population. Persistent nephrogenic cell rests (nodular renal blastema) and nephroblastomatosis are non-malignant pathological entities which reflect abnormal development of a similar cell population. The median age at diagnosis is 3.5 years, but occasionally older children, or even adults, are affected.

There is a characteristic association between Wilms' tumour, aniridia and hemihypertrophy of trunk and limbs. Several other genito-urinary anomalies may occur, including extrophic bladder, imperforate anus, ectopic ureter and hyperspadias. The frequency of aniridia in Wilms' tumour is approximately 1:100 compared with 1:50 000 for the general population, in whom it may occur sporadically or be inherited in an autosomal dominant manner. The relationship between Wilms' tumour and chromosome 11 abnormalities has been previously described (Chapter 3).

The Drash syndrome is an association between Wilms' tumour and nephritis, with or without pseudohermaphroditism. Renal failure almost

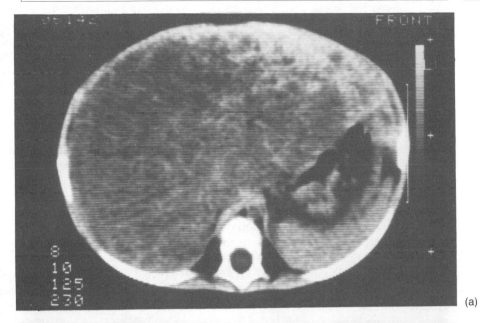

(a)

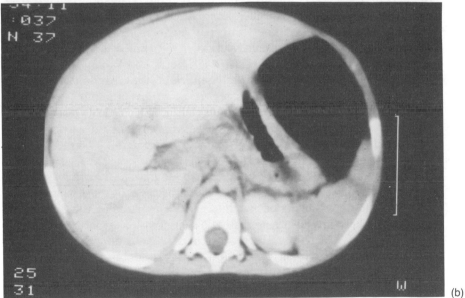

(b)

Figure 9.16 Marked hepatic enlargement associated with tumour infiltration in an infant with stage 4(s) neuroblastoma (a) and two years later after observation only (b).

invariably develops and transplantation may be appropriate once the Wilms' tumour is cured (Drash *et al.*, 1970). Beckwith's syndrome, a congenital condition with organomegaly, macroglossia, hemihypertrophy and exomphalos, has a high incidence of Wilms' tumour in addition to renal medullary hyperplasia, hepatoblastoma and adrenal carcinoma. The question often arises as to the need for regular screening of children with aniridia or Beckwith's syndrome; with the latter the risk of Wilms' tumour may be as high as 25%. Three to six monthly ultrasound examinations have been recommended, but such an approach engenders considerable parental anxiety and there is little evidence that tumours are picked up significantly earlier or that it influences the likelihood of cure. A high index of suspicion is probably sufficient in such cases after an initial ultrasound has shown normal kidneys (Azouz *et al.*, 1990).

The pathological sub-classification of Wilms' tumour is one of the more useful and internationally standardized systems and of considerable prognostic value. This is largely due to the extensive work by the American National Wilms' Tumour Study Group. Two broad prognostic groups have been ascertained, 'favourable' and 'unfavourable'. The favourable group comprises about 90% of patients in whom there is evidence of three cell sub-types (triphasic): blastemal, epithelial and stromal. The unfavourable sub-group is either anaplastic or sarcomatous. The latter includes the clear cell sarcoma, with particular propensity to metastasize to bone (Marsden, Lawler and Kumar, 1978) and the rhabdoid brain metastasizing tumour (Weeks *et al.*, 1989; Berry and Vujanic, 1992). Due to its chemoresistance and clinical behaviour the rhabdoid tumour is increasingly excluded from the category of Wilms' tumour. Congenital mesoblastic nephroma is a rare spindle cell tumour, which presents as an abdominal mass, often in the neonate and which, since it carries only a very small risk of metastases, is generally treated by surgery alone (Steinfeld *et al.*, 1984).

Wilms' tumours usually present as an abdominal mass. A babysitter or grandparent may notice the swelling which because of its slow evolution and the general well being of the child has been missed by the parents. In most cases there are few or no systemic symptoms. Haematuria occurs in only 10–15% of patients. Hypertension is seen in approximately 10% and may be due to renin production by the tumour or renal vascular compression. About one-fifth of patients show some low-grade intermittent fever.

Initial clinical examination may give a clue to operability. A mobile, well circumscribed mass without nodal or retroperitoneal extension may be resectable despite its great size. An initial IVP may be done to demonstrate the presence of a normal contralateral kidney, although ultrasound has now replaced this. The ultrasound confirms the organ of origin and will give information on nodal involvement or liver secondaries.

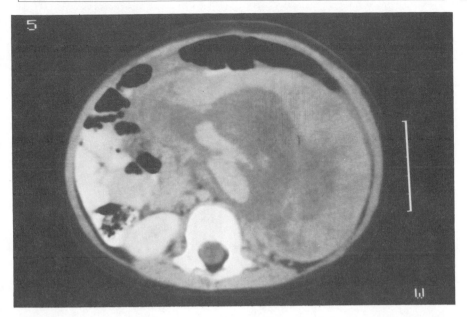

Figure 9.17 CT scan of the abdomen showing a massive left-sided Wilms' tumour with the typical venous lake appearance.

Using Doppler ultrasound vena caval involvement can be determined. CT scan is, however, advisable for accurate preoperative assessment (Figure 9.17).

Contra-indications to primary surgery include an extensively infiltrating tumour, inferior vena caval involvement or any distant metastases. Chest X-ray is mandatory to exclude lung deposits (Figure 9.18). The role of CT lung scan remains controversial, as it may upstage otherwise stage I patients and lead to possibly excessive chemotherapy and irradiation (Green *et al.*, 1991).

There is a recent tendency to use preoperative chemotherapy more frequently. This is because almost invariably the chemosensitivity of the tumour leads to simpler surgical procedures and a lower risk of tumour rupture into the peritoneal cavity (Lemerle *et al.*, 1983). Some groups, such as SIOP, recommend routine preoperative chemotherapy. If no pretreatment biopsy is performed a wrong clinical diagnosis will be made in about 5% of patients and will include a small number of benign tumours. It is therefore current policy in the UK that all tumours are biopsied if there is not to be an initial nephrectomy. If this shows clear cell tumour, a bone scan is done to exclude metastases and with the rhabdoid sub-group a head CT scan is performed. If possible, preoperative

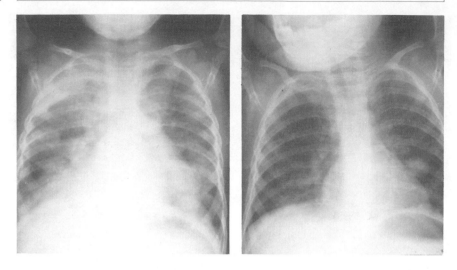

Figure 9.18 Chest X-ray in a child with multiple metastatic lesions before and following chemotherapy.

catecholamine assays should be estimated to exclude intrarenal neuro-blastoma, as this may be associated with severe intraoperative hyper-tension. A percutaneous needle biopsy is usually sufficient for initial diagnosis of inoperable cases and as these children will be receiving intensive chemotherapy there is not felt to be any significant risk of tumour spread by such a procedure. The NWTS staging system is shown in Table 9.15.

In most protocols cyclophosphamide has been omitted because it has not been shown to increase effectiveness and carries the risk of sterilizing these highly curable children (D'Angio *et al.*, 1989). In stage I disease a short course of vincristine is given and for other stages combinations of vincristine, actinomycin D and doxorubicin are used (Table 9.16). Irradiation to the tumour bed is limited to those with initially unresectable disease who have incomplete resection after chemotherapy and some patients with unfavourable histology. Lung irradiation is often given where there are pulmonary metastases, but the need for this in chemo-sensitive tumours remains debatable (DeKraker *et al.*, 1990). Cure rates with stage II disease exceed 80%; even with initially unresectable tumours, 5-year survival is around 75% and with metastatic disease (usually to lung) this is ~60%.

In about 5% of cases there is bilateral disease at presentation (Coppes *et al.*, 1989). Management of such patients requires close co-operation between oncologist and paediatric surgeon. The aim is to shrink both

Table 9.15 The National Wilms' Tumour Study Group staging of Wilms' tumours

Stage	Definitions and comments
I	**Tumour limited to the kidney and completely excised** The renal capsule is intact. The tumour has not ruptured nor been punctured before its excision. No tumour is observed in the renal bed, and histological examination confirms that the capsule is intact
II	**Tumour extends outside the kidney, but is completely excised** There is a local extension of the tumour, in particular: – penetration of the tumour into the perirenal tissues beyond the false capsule of the tumour and 'adhesions' are confirmed histologically to be due to tumour – Invasion of the para-aortic nodes, confirmed histologically; the pathologist must make a careful search of all the excised nodes for foci of tumour cells – Invasion of the renal vessel walls outside the kidney or thrombosis caused by tumour in these vessels. Thrombosis which is apparently non-neoplastic may contain islands of tumour cells, thrombi must be examined very carefully – Invasion of the renal pelvis and ureter
III	**Incomplete excision, without haematogenous metastases** This stage has been reached if one or several of the following conditions are present: – Tumour rupture before or during surgery – Peritoneal metastases, as distinguished from the simple tumour adhesions of stage II – Invasion of lymph nodes beyond the abdominal periaortic nodes – Complete excision impossible (e.g. infiltration of the vena cava)
IV	**Haematogenous metastases** Involving lung, liver, bones, brain etc.
V	**Bilateral renal tumours**

Table 9.16 Wilms' tumour chemotherapy (favourable histology)

Stage I	Vincristine weekly × 10
Stage II	Vincristine, actinomycin 3 weekly × 6/12
Stage III	Vincristine + alternating actinomycin + doxorubicin 3 weekly × 12/12
Stage IV	Vincristine + simultaneous actinomycin + doxorubicin × 12/12

Stages III and IV resect primary tumour after 3–4 months chemotherapy.
Irradiate only if residual disease at this time.
Lung irradiation in stage IV if not in CR on CT after 12 weeks

lesions maximally with chemotherapy and then perform partial nephrec-
tomies with conservation of as much normal renal tissue as possible. With
this approach ~75% of patients should be cured and adequate renal
function preserved.

9.6 SOFT TISSUE SARCOMAS

The commonest soft tissue sarcoma in childhood is the rhabdomyosarcoma. This tumour arises from embryonal striated muscle precursor
cells which proliferate to produce a variety of morphological forms.
The two commonest groups are the embryonal and the alveolar type.
The former consists mainly of small primitive spindle shaped cells with
elongated nuclei. The characteristic feature of the alveolar form is the
micro-architecture which resembles pulmonary alveoli, lined by rounded,
sometimes multinucleate cells. This sub-division has prognostic significance, with the alveolar group which often occurs on limbs and in
older children, doing poorly (Reboul-Marty *et al.*, 1991; Rodary *et al.*,
1991). A further sub-group within embryonal rhabdomyosarcoma is the
botryoid form, so called because of its tendency to form mucosa-lined,
grape-like masses occurring in hollow viscera such as the vagina, bladder
or auditory canal. This group has a particularly good outcome (Maurer
et al., 1988; Newton *et al.*, 1988). A third, pleomorphic or adult, form is
rare in childhood.

About half the cases of rhabdomyosarcoma occur in the head and

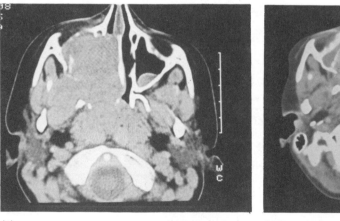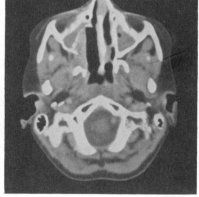

(a)   (b)

Figure 9.19 (a) Primary tumour arising in the nasopharyngeal region with extensive tumour infiltration through the nasal septi and infraorbital bones. (b) Following chemotherapy there is dramatic resolution with some bony reconstruction.

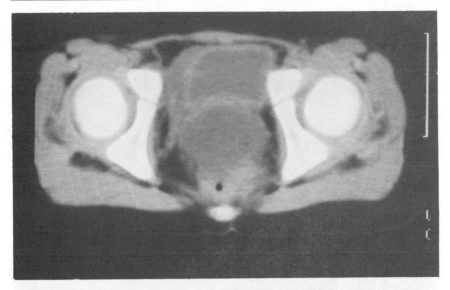

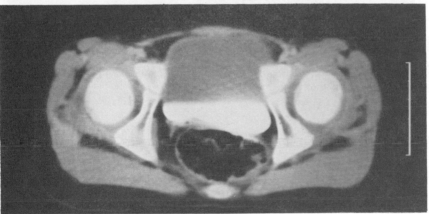

Figure 9.20 Rhabdomyosarcoma arising posterior to the bladder which is filled with urine (top). Following chemotherapy there is no evidence of tumour residue (bottom).

neck region such as orbit, nasopharynx, middle ear and face (Figure 9.19). A quarter affect the genito-urinary system, involving the bladder, prostate, vagina, uterus or paratesticular region (Figure 9.20), and the remainder involve the extremities (Figure 9.21), trunk or retroperitoneum. Lesions of the head and neck can present as superficial swellings, but may extend into the facial bones, causing bony and cartilaginous destruction. There may be intracranial extension or involvement of the

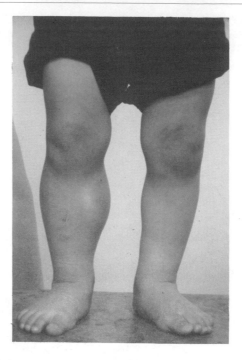

Figure 9.21 Rhabdomyosarcoma of the right calf. The mass is clearly seen compared to the normal left leg.

base of the skull, producing cranial nerve palsy. Nasopharyngeal lesions often present with nasal obstruction or bloodstained mucous discharge. Orbital tumours cause proptosis and strabismus and occasionally are localized to the conjunctiva. Orbital lesions may be misdiagnosed as cysts, orbital cellulitis or an idiopathic squint. Bladder tumours can cause dysuria, haematuria, strangury or present as an abdominal mass. Blood-stained vaginal discharge is usually the first sign of the botryoid vaginal tumour. Limb lesions are usually painless. Disseminated alveolar rhabdomyosarcoma with marrow involvement can present with symptomatic hypercalcaemia and DIC.

Staging investigations should include chest X-ray and CT scan; abdominal CT for abdominal and pelvic lesions and head scan for head and neck lesions. Technetium bone scan and bone marrow aspirate and biopsy should also be performed. Various different staging systems are used (Tables 9.17, 9.18), but the local extent of tumour, i.e. regional or localized, appears to be of major prognostic significance (Kingston, McElwain and Malpas, 1983; Lawrence *et al.*, 1987; Rodary, Flamant and Donaldson, 1989). Localized disease can usually be completely resected

Table 9.17 American IRS grouping system

Group I	Localised disease, completely resected Confined to organ or muscle of origin Infiltration outside organ or muscle of origin; regional nodes not involved
Group II	Regional disease, grossly resected A. Grossly resected tumours with microscopic residue B. Regional disease, completely resected, in which nodes may be involved and/or extension of tumour into an adjacent organ present C. Regional disease with involved nodes, grossly resected, but with evidence of microscopic residue
Group III	Incomplete resection or biopsy with gross residual disease
Group IV	Distant metastases present at onset

Table 9.18 TNM staging system

T1	Tumour confined to organ or tissue of origin
1a	5 cm or less in size
1b	more than 3 cm in size
T2	Tumour involves contiguous organs or structures
2a	5 cm or less in size
2b	more than 5 cm in size
N0	No clinical or radiographic evidence of involvement of regional lymph nodes (no histologic determination)
N1	Clinical or radiographic evidence of regional lymph node involvement
M0	No distant metastases on clinical, radiographic, or bone marrow assessment
M1	Evidence of distant metastasis

European SIOP staging system

Clinic stage	Invasiveness	Size	Nodal status	Metastasis status
I	T1	a or b	N0	M0
II	T2	a or b	N0	M0
III	T1 or T2	a or b	N1	M0
IV	T1 or T2	a or b	N0 or N1	M1

either at presentation or following chemotherapy. With regional disease there is often microscopic residue postsurgery unless unacceptably radical resection is involved. Sites with a particularly good prognosis are the orbit, paratesticular region, vagina and bladder (Table 9.19). The poorest prognostic group remain those with parameningeal lesions (i.e. naso-

Table 9.19 Four-year survival rates by prognostic groups (primary site and extent)

Primary site	% of patients	4-year survival rate (%) T_1	T_2
Orbit	10	90	85
Head and neck	12	80	50
Parameningeal	17	60	50
Bladder, prostate	13	80	50
Other genitourinary sites	15	95	60
Limbs	13	60	40
Other	20	50	45

pharynx, paranasal sinuses, middle ear and base of skull) in whom local surgical control is particularly difficult and there are high rates of local recurrence, sometimes with meningeal involvement. Patients with metastatic disease also do badly, in particular those with bone marrow involvement.

In the past, the treatment approach was to give standard dose chemotherapy combined with aggressive surgery and early wide field irradiation, except where the tumour was completely resected at presentation when radiotherapy was omitted (Crist *et al.*, 1990). This approach has been challenged by many European groups, who place greater emphasis on the role of initial intensive chemotherapy. This is designed to reduce both the rate of metastatic relapse and the sometimes considerable long-term morbidity of high-dose radiotherapy to growing bones, or the sequelae of radical surgery. With this approach, unless the primary tumour is localized and readily resectable, initial surgery is limited to biopsy alone. Chemotherapy is then given to achieve maximal tumour shrinkage (usually 4–6 months). If complete remission is achieved by this approach, and where possible proven by second-look surgery, then no irradiation is given (Flamant *et al.*, 1991). This applies to all stages of disease and although local control using this approach may be somewhat inferior to that using radical surgery and radiotherapy, many local recurrences are cured with second-line chemotherapy and irradiation. In certain sites, such as the nasopharynx or orbit, it is particularly difficult to prove complete remission following chemotherapy and in these cases if initially there has been bony erosion or is any suspicious lesion on CT scan after chemotherapy, irradiation should be given.

Chemotherapy combinations usually comprise cyclophosphamide or ifosfamide, vincristine and actinomycin D or adriamycin (Table 9.20). Newer agents such as etoposide and possibly cisplatin or carboplatin may also be effective (Miser *et al.*, 1987; Phillips and Pinkerton, 1992). Because

Table 9.20 Treatment strategy in rhabdomyosarcoma

Localized, resectable tumour		
Surgery	if complete	VA × 10/52
	incomplete	IVA × 4 courses
Regional, unresectable tumour		
Primary chemotherapy		IVA or VACA
		× 4–6 courses depending on site
Delayed surgery		
Irradiate if no CR achieved or		
parameningeal with bone erosion		
Metastatic		
More intensive multidrug regimen, e.g. add platinum–etoposide		
? megatherapy with marrow rescue		

VA   = vincristine, actinomycin
IVA = ifosfamide, vincristine, actinomycin
VACA = vincristine, actinomycin, cyclophosphamide, adriamycin

of the poor prognosis for patients with metastatic disease the role of very high dose therapy with autologous bone marrow rescue is currently under evaluation (Pinkerton *et al.*, 1991).

Treatment approaches for rhabdomyosarcoma are tailored toward the site involved and also to the age and growth potential of the patient (King and Clatworthy, 1981).

Orbital tumours can be readily cured with external beam irradiation and a short course of conventional chemotherapy. There is, however, concern about the effect on growth of periorbital bone in the younger child and also lack of tears, entropion and cataracts. Using careful radiotherapy techniques, these sequelae may be minimal but it is likely that in patients with highly chemosensitive tumours who achieve a complete response radiotherapy may not be required (Rousseau *et al.*, 1992).

With parameningeal primaries, some centres treat the whole brain with 25–30 Gy and boost the primary site up to 55 Gy. In addition, intrathecal chemotherapy has been given. This aggressive approach may not be necessary and patients given intensive chemotherapy with irradiation localized to the primary site have not been shown to do significantly worse (Gasparini *et al.*, 1990). Again, there is obviously concern about the late sequelae of extended field high-dose irradiation (Heyn *et al.*, 1986).

In the urogenital system the paratesticular rhabdomyosarcoma do particularly well, partly due to the surgical accessibility of the tumour (Raney *et al.*, 1978; Hamilton, 1989). Nodal involvement should be carefully excluded by CT scanning but lymph node resection is not necessary (Olive *et al.*, 1984). If complete remission is achieved with chemotherapy alone, irradiation is not required. With tumours of the bladder, prostate, vagina and uterus, the radical surgical approach has now been largely replaced by more aggressive initial chemotherapy. In this way bladder-conserving surgery may be possible, either by retaining as much normal bladder as possible but ensuring clear margins of excision, or by partial cystectomy with preservation of the trigone region for later reconstructive surgery (Raney *et al.*, 1990).

Small volume residual disease may be treatable with interstitial radiotherapy techniques rather than external beam irradiation. Iridium wires are inserted directly into the tissue or in the case of the vagina a plastic mould may be constructed to carry the radioactive source (Flamant *et al.*, 1990) (Figure 7.1).

The ultimate aim of these approaches is to improve cosmetic and functional outcome where possible, but not at the cost of any reduction in cure rate. With most treatment regimens 5-year survival for completely resected, localized disease should exceed 80%. For regional disease where complete remission is achieved with chemotherapy alone or combined with surgery or radiotherapy for minimal residual disease, 5-year survival should approach 70%, with the exception of high-risk parameningeal primaries and alveolar histology. For metastatic disease, long-term survival remains less than 25% (Koscielniak *et al.*, 1992).

Other rare sarcomas include fibrosarcoma, synovial sarcoma, liposarcoma and neurofibrosarcoma. These tend to be less chemosensitive

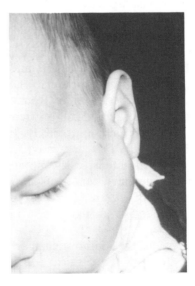

Figure 9.22 An infantile fibrosarcoma arising in the left preauricular region.

than rhabdomyosarcoma and consequently surgery plays a more important role in management (Gasparini and Lombardi, 1986; Horowitz *et al.*, 1986).

Infantile fibrosarcoma and fibromatosis may respond to low-dose chemotherapy such as vincristine and actinomycin with gradual tumour shrinkage, allowing eventual surgical excision (Figure 9.22).

9.7 BONE SARCOMAS

Osteogenic sarcoma is the commonest primary bone tumour in children, with a median onset of 12 years. The age distribution suggests an association with a period of rapid growth and the high incidence in weight-bearing lower limb bones may be of significance. Osteosarcomas may be due to irradiation and in the past, jaw tumours were described in painters of luminous watch dials due to licking radioactive paintbrush tips. More recently, radiotherapy for soft tissue sarcoma or retinoblastoma has been implicated. In retinoblastoma there is the risk to orbital bone if irradiated but also an increased incidence in distant bones suggesting an inherent predisposition.

By definition, osteogenic sarcoma has a sarcomatous stroma and formation of osteoid or bone. Pathological subdivisions reflect the predominant cell type, i.e. fibroblastic, chondroblastic or osteoblastic. The rare, highly undifferentiated small cell osteosarcoma may be difficult to distinguish from other small round cell tumours. Subgroups are also based on radiological features: medullary, arising in the medullary cavity in the metaphyseal region and passing through the cortex beneath the periosteum; telangiectatic, a purely osteolytic lesion, predominantly cystic and necrotic; periosteal, located in the bony cortex without extension into the medullary cavity but sometimes with extensive soft tissue involvement. The periosteal tumour is usually of high-grade malignancy, unlike the paraosteal form where tumour arises in the cortex and, attached by a broad base, may encircle the bone. With paraosteal variety there is no soft tissue infiltration and the tumour is well differentiated with highly formed osteoid. For the parasteal tumour surgery alone is adequate, in contrast with all the other forms which have high metastatic potential and therefore require systemic chemotherapy.

The commonest presentation is localized pain, with or without swelling (Figure 9.23). The latter may be quite marked without significant pain but there is usually some reduction in normal function and pathological fractures may occur (Figure 9.24). The commonest sites for osteosarcoma are femur (50%), tibia (30%) and humerus (10%). Plain X-ray shows evidence of soft tissue involvement in three-quarters of patients. The bone lesion usually has a mixed lytic/osteoblastic component, but in 20%

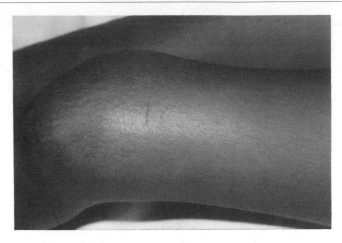

Figure 9.23 A swollen tender left knee due to an osteosarcoma of the lower femur.

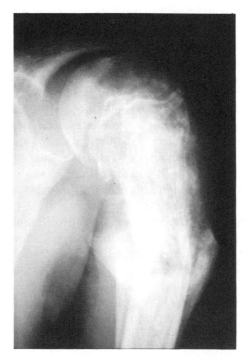

Figure 9.24 Pathological fracture of upper humerus due to osteogenic sarcoma. The extensive soft tissue calcification within the mass is clearly seen.

it is purely lytic or blastic. Differential diagnosis includes osteomyelitis; traumatic fracture; metastatic lesions, such as neuroblastoma; lymphoma and eosinophilic granuloma. Benign lesions, such as osteoma and chondroma generally have more clearly defined edges on X ray.

Biopsy is essential for the diagnosis of osteosarcoma and this should be done through a small skin site which can be excised at the time of the definitive surgery. Staging studies include chest X-ray with CT scan if negative and technetium bone scan, to detect bony metastases or the rare polyostotic form. CT scan or MRI scan will delineate the extent of soft tissue involvement and of intramedullary extension. As in Ewing's sarcoma the MRI may be particularly useful in this role (MacVicar et al., 1992).

In the management of osteosarcoma close cooperation between the oncologist and the orthopaedic surgeon is required so that the timing and type of surgery is optimal, both in terms of cancer control and functional outcome.

In the pre-chemotherapy era amputation, with or without local irradiation, at best produced long-term relapse-free survival of 20%. Figures as high as 50% with surgery alone have been published, but this improvement over similarly treated historical controls may reflect patient selection. Studies using 'adjuvant chemotherapy' given after amputation showed a reduction in metastatic relapse rates (Goorin et al., 1987). The concept of preoperative chemotherapy was subsequently developed and has the advantage of achieving tumour reduction prior to surgery, thus facilitating conservative limb-preserving procedures. It was suggested that the response to initial chemotherapy correlated with ultimate prognosis and in the case of a poor response, outcome could be improved by altering the chemotherapy regimen. This concept, however, remains unproven (Rosen et al., 1982).

Randomised trials have now demonstrated clearly that both relapse-free survival and overall survival are significantly improved by adjuvant chemotherapy using regimens including doxorubicin, cisplatin and high-dose methotrexate (Link et al., 1986; Eilber et al., 1987). Intra-arterial chemotherapy has been used to try to increase effective drug concentration in tumour but is of unproven value (Jaffe et al., 1985).

The surgical approach has also changed over recent years. Amputation with excision of the entire bone was the standard approach in the past. With effective preoperative chemotherapy there is an increasing trend towards en bloc resection of tumour, with limb preservation (Figure 9.25). There must, however, be at least 8 cm of tumour-free bone either side of the resection and the residual soft tissue extension should be minimal. Amputation at presentation remains the treatment of choice for a very large lesion, particularly if there is infection or a pathological fracture.

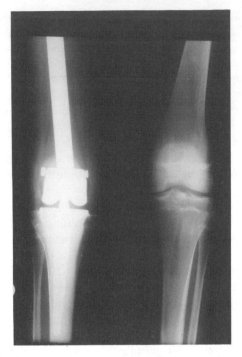

Figure 9.25 Prosthetic replacement of lower femur and knee joint following chemotherapy and *en bloc* resection of lower femoral osteosarcoma.

Patients who are suitable for limb preservation must be carefully selected and early cosmetic result should not be the sole end point. In children who still have several centimetres of growth, the long-term result may be poor due to marked limb shortening. If this is only a few centimetres then adjustable prostheses which may be lengthened with time are a possibility. Alternatively the epiphysis on the contralateral leg may be stapled to prevent growth. With tibial tumours, where most of the proximal bone may be resected, there is often difficulty in finding attachment for muscles around the knee which results in poor function. For these reasons, amputation with early mobilization may be the treatment of choice. Children quickly adapt to detachable limb prostheses and after a short period acquire remarkable agility.

Where a limb-conserving approach is chosen, a variety of options are available. These include metal prostheses for knee, shoulder or elbow joints and autologous bone grafts, e.g. fibula replacing the humerus. Allogeneic bone grafts from cadavers, with insertion of long sections of bone may be possible. Bone grafting often requires prolonged immobilization and moreover there remains a significant risk of ultimately requiring amputation. An unusual but effective approach for lower femur or upper tibia lesions is the rotationplasty. The nerves and vessels are preserved and the foot is re-grafted onto the stump, facing posteriorly. Inserted in a detachable limb prosthesis, this provides greater control than a conventional stump.

Metastatic disease at presentation is the single most important adverse prognostic sign (Figure 9.26). This is most commonly lung or bone and the latter has a particularly poor outlook. Lung irradiation plays no role in the management of lung metastases and has no prophylactic value. Young age is an adverse factor and it has been shown that hyperdiploid DNA content in tumour cells is associated with poor outcome (Look *et al.*, 1988).

Osteosarcoma is one tumour where surgery has an important role in the management of pulmonary metastases. Resection of secondary deposits which remain after chemotherapy may improve survival. In the case of isolated pulmonary relapse resection of the lesions may be curative (Rosenberg *et al.*, 1979). It is, however, normal practice to give second-line chemotherapy to assess chemosensitivity prior to surgery.

Chondrosarcomas are very rare in children, but may arise in pre-existing osteochondroma or enchondroma. These do not tend to metastasize and treatment is surgical.

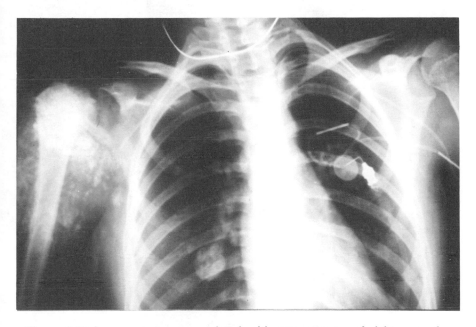

Figure 9.26 Lung metastases associated with osteosarcoma of right upper humerus. An intra-arterial catheter is in place for administration of intra-tumoral chemotherapy.

Ewing's sarcoma

The cellular origin of Ewing's sarcoma of bone remains obscure, and was originally thought to be from vascular endothelium. There is a current trend to group this tumour with the primitive neuroectodermal tumours with which it shares a characteristic t(11;22) translocation (Jurgens *et al.*, 1988b).

Ewing's sarcoma is composed of a diffuse, structureless infiltration of small round cells with irregular, rounded or oval nuclei and slightly granular cytoplasm. Mitotic activity is not particularly prominent. Characteristically the tumour is PAS and reticulin positive in the strands of fibrous tissue between groups of tumour cells. Because of the lack of specific pathological features, the diagnosis is largely based on the tumour site, and by exclusion of other small round cell tumours.

The tumour typically presents with local bony pain or swelling or soft tissue extension. Fever occurs in about a third of patients. The diaphyseal region is typically involved unlike osteosarcoma where the lesion is usually epiphyseal. The sites most commonly involved are the pelvis,

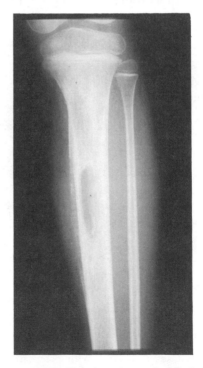

Figure 9.27 Plain X-ray of tibia showing the typical lytic lesion of Ewing's sarcoma. There is also some periosteal elevation and soft tissue swelling.

the femur, humerus and rib. Iliac primaries may be associated with an extensive soft tissue mass presenting as an abdominal mass. Paravertebral lesions may present with focal weakness. There is metastatic disease at presentation in ca. 25% involving lung, bone, bone marrow or pleura.

Plain X-ray will show diaphyseal tumour extending along to the metaphysis. The lesion can be lytic or mixed lytic sclerotic and may be lamellated with new bone formation. About two-thirds have a soft tissue mass and pathological fractures are sometimes seen (Figure 9.27).

Initial staging investigations to detect metastatic disease include technetium bone scan and CT scan of lungs. Bone marrow aspirate and trephine should be done in all patients with bulky primary disease. CT scan of primary disease in long bones may give information about the degree of soft tissue involvement and the disease in the medullary cavity both pre- and post-chemotherapy. MRI may demonstrate extensive unexpected disease at these sites. This may be of particular importance in planning limb preserving surgery as the margins of excision must be well clear of any residual tumour (MacVicker et al., 1992) (Figure 9.28).

In the young child a urinary catecholamine evaluation is mandatory to exclude neuroblastoma.

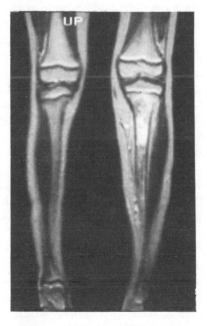

Figure 9.28 Magnetic resonance image of Ewing's sarcoma (same tumour as in Figure 9.27). With this imaging modality the tumour is seen to extend up to the epiphysial plate and into the adjacent soft tissue.

Table 9.21 Treatment strategy in bone tumours

Primary chemotherapy
   Doxorubicin–cisplatin (osteosarcoma)
   Ifosfamide, vincristine, doxorubicin (IVAd) or vincristine, actinomycin,
   cyclophosphamide, adriamycin (VACA) (Ewing's)

Delayed surgery after 12–16 weeks
   Resection with prosthesis or amputation

Continued chemotherapy
   6/12 total in osteosarcoma
   9/12–12/12 total in Ewing's

Radiation used as alternative to surgery in Ewing's sarcoma

Lung metastases are resected after primary chemotherapy in osteosarcoma.
Lung irradiation is rarely used with either osteosarcoma or Ewing's

With surgery alone overall survival was 15% and radiotherapy alone around 10%. Combined with effective systemic chemotherapy such as combinations of vincristine, actinomycin D, doxorubicin and cyclophosphamide or ifosfamide, cure rates for lesions of small volume and particularly at distal sites is over 60%. With large volume lesions, especially in the pelvis, where the radiation dose may be limited by intestinal toxicity and surgical resection is difficult, the outcome remains poor (10–20% long-term survival). The presence of metastases at diagnosis and the degree of soft tissue extension also influences prognosis. Treatment strategy depends upon the site and size of tumour. A small tumour in an expendable bone, such as metatarsal or fibula, may be resected as a primary procedure. In general, however, chemotherapy is given and once tumour shrinkage has been achieved local treatment with non-deforming surgery or radiotherapy is carried out (Jurgens *et al.*, 1988a; Burgert *et al.*, 1990).

New drug combinations, alternative drug scheduling and the use of megatherapy procedures are currently under evaluation for bad risk patients and there is a trend towards more aggressive surgery to improve local control.

The term PNET (primitive neuroectodermal tumours) encompasses a group of tumours also called peripheral neuroepithelioma. Unfortunately this term PNET is also used for a medulloblastoma-like tumour that arises outside the cerebellum. The terms peripheral and cranial PNET are appropriate to distinguish these two entities which differ both pathologically and biologically. It is likely that the soft tissue (or non-osseous) Ewing's is part of the spectrum of peripheral PNETs and shares the typical t(11;22). When a peripheral PNET arises in the chest wall it is sometimes called an Askin tumour. They may, however, occur at almost any soft tissue site and are usually treated like a rhabdomyosarcoma (Kinsella *et al.*, 1983; Jurgens *et al.*, 1988b).

9.8 LIVER TUMOURS

Primary liver tumours in children are usually either hepatocarcinoma or hepatoblastoma. Sarcomas, such as rhabdomyosarcoma and angiosarcoma are also occasionally seen. Benign lesions include haemangioma, hamartoma and adenoma.

Hepatoblastoma is an embryonal tumour arising in primitive hepatocytes. It usually presents in infancy and is rare over 5 years of age. Histologically there are three subgroups, the fetal type with cells resembling those found in the perinatal liver, the embryonal type with a rather more primitive structure and the anaplastic, highly undifferentiated form.

In hepatocarcinoma the tumour cells resemble those seen in adult disease and there may occasionally be a history of associated liver cirrhosis.

The presenting sign is often an abdominal mass and with marked distension. Pain is unusual but there may be a history of anorexia and vomiting. Plain X-ray can show calcification and ultrasound usually reveals the liver to be the site of origin. CT scan will delineate the extent of the primary tumour which is of major importance when deciding on initial therapy, particularly operability (Finn *et al.*, 1990).

Elevation of serum alpha-fetoprotein (AFP) is a useful marker for hepatoblastoma and this is also elevated in about half the patients with hepatic carcinoma. This glycoprotein is produced in fetal yolk sac, liver and intestine. It reaches maximum levels at 13 weeks' gestation and falls to adult levels ($<10\,\mu$g/ml) within the first three months.

Initial staging investigations for liver tumours include CT scan of chest and abdomen and technetium bone scan.

Completeness of surgery is the most important single prognostic factor with these tumours but because of the extent of the lesion operative mortality may be high. About 60% of patients with localized, resectable hepatoblastoma will be cured (Siegel *et al.*, 1980). This is, however, a highly chemosensitive tumour and therefore adjuvant chemotherapy with doxorubicin alone is given to patients with completely resected disease. Where the primary is considered unresectable more intensive regimens, including doxorubicin and cisplatin (Ortego, 1989) are given and surgery delayed until the AFP is normal or maximally reduced and CT scan indicates operability (Figure 9.29). At this time angiography and MRI may have a useful role in planning surgery. The serum AFP level is a

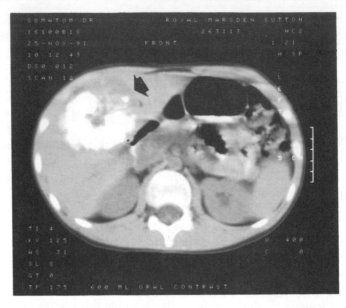

Figure 9.29 CT scan of hepatoblastoma showing extensive calcification following PLADO chemotherapy.

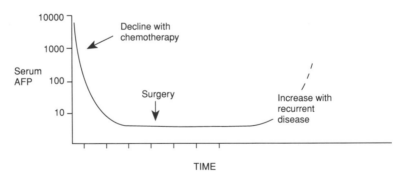

Figure 9.30 AFP pattern during therapy and follow-up in hepatoblastoma.

useful guide to response to chemotherapy as it should decline with a half-life of 5–7 days. It may also be an early clue to disease relapse (Figure 9.30).

Haemangioma or haemangio-endothelioma of the liver, although not malignant diseases, may produce considerable management problems due to high output cardiac failure or consumptive thrombocytopenia. Vascular embolization is often successful, but in some cases there may be a role for external beam irradiation or sarcoma-type chemotherapy.

9.9 RETINOBLASTOMA

Retinoblastoma is a tumour of neuroectodermal origin arising in retinal tissue. Sixty per cent of cases involve only one eye; in the remainder the lesions are bilateral and in the rare trilateral form there is an additional mid-line lesion in the region of the pineal or anterior end of the third ventricle. This is due to ectopic retinal tissue and is part of a multifocal primary rather than metastatic disease.

The genetics of retinoblastoma has already been discussed (Chapter 2) and its association with deletions on chromosome 13.

Clinical presentation is almost invariably at below 3 years of age and it is rare for the disease to develop later than 5 years of age. The disease is usually confined to the eye at presentation. Loss of the normal red reflex when light is shone directly into the eye indicates the presence of a space occupying lesion on the retina. Small lesions arising in the macular region may disturb vision and lead to strabismus. With multiple lesions there may be secondary glaucoma.

Spread of the tumour is initially along the optic nerve and into the spinal fluid. Rarely marrow or bone metastases are found.

Initial assessment should be under general anaesthesia to enable adequate examination of the retinal surface. In the sporadic form the tumour is almost invariably solitary whereas in the inherited form several lesions are often seen in the same eye or involving the other retina. Plain X-ray of the orbit may demonstrate calcification and similarly a calcified mass can be shown with ultrasound or CT scanning.

Differential diagnosis from infective lesions such as *Toxicara canis* can usually be made by an experienced paediatric ophthalmologist. Confirmation of diagnosis may require biopsy but this is not usually necessary particularly where there is a family history of the condition (Hungerford, Kingston and Plowman, 1986).

The treatment of retinoblastoma depends on the extent of the tumour and in general is as conservative as possible. Adverse prognostic features which preclude a conservative approach are involvement of the optic disc, which may be apparent from fundoscopy or CT scan, or where there is a high risk of heavy choroidal invasion, which accompanies either glaucoma or retinal detachment.

Focal treatment involves either xenon arc photocoagulation, radiotherapy applied by surface applicator, such as cobalt 60, or external beam radiotherapy. For the last elaborate systems have been developed using a contact lens to provide a fixed point from which all measurements are made and the linear accelerator beam is directed (Harnett *et al.*, 1987). This approach is particularly suitable for posterior solitary lesions without vitreous seeding and will avoid the inevitable cataract which develops about one to two years after standard external beam irradiation. It also prevents shrinkage of the bony orbit and eyelids which may lead to exposure keratitis and cosmetic defects.

Enucleation of the eye is now relatively uncommon, but if necessary as much of the orbital portion of the optic nerve must be excised with the eye to obtain histological confirmation regarding tumour infiltration.

Indications for adjuvant chemotherapy are the presence of optic nerve involvement and heavy choroidal involvement. Active agents include cyclophosphamide and ifosfamide and regimens used for neuroectodermal tumours at other sites may be appropriate, e.g. cisplatin–etoposide combinations (Kingston, Hungerford and Plowman, 1987).

Where the tumour is solitary and there is no family history, recurrence in the same contralateral eye is unlikely but close follow-up is none the less necessary. Examination under anaesthesia should be done every three to four months for two years and then six monthly for up to 5 years of age. These patients should be looked after in specialized units and in the UK the vast majority of children are seen in one of two centres. The survival should approach 100% in patients treated conservatively. Only about 30% survive where there is optic nerve involvement and 75% with choroidal invasion.

Where there is no previous family history and one affected child, other children incur about a 5% risk of being affected. By contrast, the offspring of a parent with bilateral disease has a 50% chance of being affected and, similarly, where a parent has had a unilateral retinoblastoma and a previous child has been affected, there is again a 50% chance of subsequent children being involved. The use of molecular genetic techniques to detect loss of heterozygosity on chromosome 13 should make the screening of high risk offspring a simpler procedure, enabling normal children to be excluded early in life and therefore avoid the very intensive ophthalmological follow-up (Yandell *et al.*, 1989). The use of antenatal screening and elective termination of affected pregnancies is somewhat controversial in view of the very high cure rates in affected children. This is clearly an individual decision for the families but many feel that the quality of life of the children and the major stress imposed on the family warrants such intervention.

Other tumours affecting the orbit include the orbital rhabdomyosarcoma, optic nerve glioma, and Langerhans' cell histiocytosis. Secondary deposits in the orbit are uncommon but may be seen with non-Hodgkin's lymphoma or lymphoblastic leukaemia. Neuroblastoma involving the orbital bones may result in marked proptosis.

9.10 HISTIOCYTIC DISORDERS

Histiocytes are a component of the mononuclear phagocytic cell system which interacts with the rest of the immune response, and plays an important role in defence against infection. Pathological entities involving the histiocyte are Langerhans' cell histiocytosis (previously known as histiocytosis X), malignant histiocytosis and the virus associated haemophagocytic syndrome.

The term Langerhans' cell histiocytosis (LCH) comprises a broad range of clinical syndromes which used to be known as eosinophilic granuloma of bone, Letterer–Siwe disease of skin and lung and Hand–Schüller–Christian disease with multisystem involvement. Because these entities all involve the same cellular abnormality and are spectrums of the same disease, they are no longer separated in this way (Broadbent and Pritchard, 1985; Chu et al., 1987).

The pathognomic feature of LCH is the presence of the Langerhans' cell, a mononuclear cell with a lobulated, grooved nucleus, uneven chromatin and eosinophilic cytoplasm. There is an associated proliferation of reactive phagocytic histiocytes, lymphocytes and polymorphs. Under the electron microscope the Langerhans' cells contain a unique racquet-shaped organelle (Burbeck granule). The cell itself does not have any phagocytic capacity, although haemophagocytosis is commonly a feature of the disease when extensive. The immunological characteristics of the Langerhans' cell have recently been clarified (Histiocyte Society Writing Group, 1987). It is important to stress that LCH is not a cancer but is frequently managed by paediatric oncologists because where treatment is necessary cytotoxic agents are often used.

LCH may be divided into two broad groups: single or multisystem disease. Single system disease often involves bone and may present with pain or a tender mass. Often asymptomatic lesions are found on routine X-ray for other reasons. The radiological features of an irregular lytic lesion with clearly defined borders are almost pathognomic, but biopsy confirmation is usually sought (Figure 9.31). This in itself may be therapeutic and induce spontaneous remission of the lesion. A skeletal survey should be done to determine the extent of the disease and although bone scans are often performed, the skeletal survey is probably more accurate for defining lesions. If there is no clinical evidence of other system involvement, i.e. no skin or lung lesions, anaemia or hepatosplenomegaly, no further staging investigations are necessary. No intervention is usually required. In the past these lesions were irradiated, but the only indications for this may be where pain is persistent despite curettage, or if there is partial collapse of a vertebral body with neurological symptoms. Complete vertebral collapse, if asymptomatic, does not benefit from irradiation.

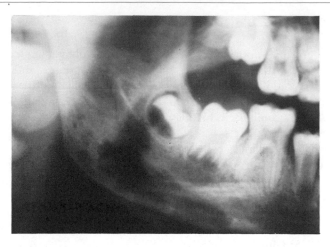

Figure 9.31 Eosinophilic granuloma of the mandible. The lytic lesion in the jaw may be associated with loosening of the teeth.

Other single system LCH involves the skin, with a seborrhoeic rash; the ears, with aural discharge or mastoid destruction; lymph nodes, with often suppurative lymphadenopathy and sinus formation (Figure 9.32).

Diabetes insipidus can result from disease involvement of the pituitary gland or hypothalamic involvement secondary to lesions in the orbit, sphenoid and mastoid. ADH status should be evaluated either by water deprivation tests or serum vasopressin levels if there is a history of polyuria or polydipsia (Dungar et al., 1989). Radiotherapy may be successful and chemotherapy can have a role.

Generalized disease involves combinations of skin, nodes, lung, bone, liver, spleen and bone marrow. The subgroup with the worst prognosis comprises infants with extensive liver, spleen and marrow involvement, often associated with extensive skin disease.

Involvement of the skull leads to large boggy soft tissue swellings with alarmingly large lytic lesions in the underlying bone. Lung involvement presents with diffuse pulmonary infiltration or honeycomb appearance.

Full staging of patients with multisystem LCH should include skeletal survey, bone marrow aspirate and trephine biopsy, chest X-ray, abdominal ultrasound, liver function tests and lung function tests (if old enough). Skin biopsy will usually show the characteristic cellular infiltrate.

Management of multisystem disease depends on the extent and the symptoms caused. The disease may be relatively indolent and little inter-

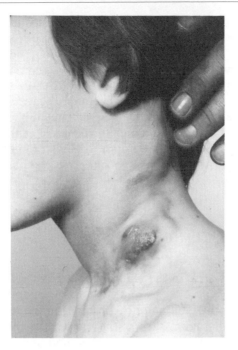

Figure 9.32 Nodal disease in Langerhan's cell histiocytosis associated with skin ulceration and recurring suppurative infection.

vention required, but with severe skin involvement or mastoid disease prednisolone and vincristine are usually first line agents. Topical treatment of severe skin disease with mustine has been successful. With refractory disease or the extensive multiorgan involvement of infants, more aggressive chemotherapy with the addition of other drugs such as etoposide may be necessary. With infant multisystem LCH there remains a significant septic mortality due to myelosuppression from marrow involvement or generalised debility (McLelland *et al.*, 1990).

Malignant histiocytosis is a rare malignant proliferation of histiocytic cells which presents with lymphadenopathy and striking systemic malaise, such as recurring fever and weight loss. Bone marrow involvement also occurs and this condition is usually treated as a high-grade lymphoma (Tseng *et al.*, 1984). With refinements in immunohistochemistry it is likely that many cases of malignant histiocytosis would now be classified as K1 positive large cell anaplastic lymphoma, usually of T-cell origin (i.e. not a true histiocytic neoplasm).

The virus-associated haemophagocytic syndrome is an abnormal pathological response to a variety of infections, including herpes simplex, varicella, CMV and EBV and adenovirus. In this condition there may be extensive liver and spleen infiltration and prominent haemophagocytosis in bone marrow. Langerhans' cells are not seen. The disease is usually self-limiting but may respond to steroids or, in severe cases, agents such as methotrexate and etoposide (Risdall *et al.*, 1979).

There is also a familial form of haemophagocytic syndrome, where there is no evidence of a preceding viral infection, often a history of previously affected infants and a high incidence of central nervous system involvement with monocytic infiltration of spinal fluid. This condition is frequently fatal but may respond to intensive chemotherapy (Alvarado *et al.*, 1986).

9.11 GERM CELL TUMOURS

Germ cell tumours arise in the pluripotential germ cell population which in fetal life normally migrates from the yolk sac endoderm to the genital ridge. The tumour may therefore occur either in the testes or ovary or in sites of aberrant migration, such as the sacrococcygeal area, retroperitoneum, mediastinum and pineal region. The undifferentiated unipotential

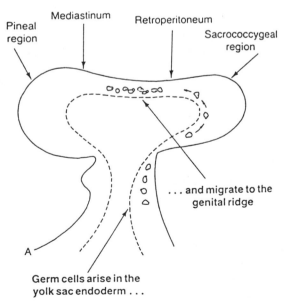

Figure 9.33 Diagrammatic representation of the origin and migration of germ cell from yolk sac to gonadal ridge, showing possible aberrant sites of migration.

primitive germ cell gives rise to a germinoma, either seminoma or dys-germinoma. The multipotential cell population which would normally contribute to the embryo or extra-embryonal structures gives rise re-spectively to teratomas and trophoblastic or yolk sac tumour (Figure 9.33). Malignant germ cell tumours in children tend to have histological features which contain two cell populations; the yolk sac tumour pro-ducing alpha-fetoprotcin and the trophoblastic tumour producing beta-HCG (human choriogonadotrophin). Pure teratomas are usually benign, although they may contain sub-populations of malignant yolk sac or trophoblastic cells. The germinoma is composed of nests of large uniform neoplastic cells with vesicular nuclei and clear cytoplasm. The yolk sac tumour typically shows a reticulated pattern with a lacy framework and contains rosettes of cells (Schiller–Duval bodies). AFP may be demon-strable in the cytoplasm of individual tumour cells. The benign, highly differentiated teratoma is often cystic and contains various somatic com-ponents such as bone, cartilage, hair and glandular structures (Dehner, 1986).

Testicular teratoma (orchioblastoma)

These usually develop as a painless scrotal swelling, or if there is exten-sive nodal involvement, as abdominal pain and a palpable mass. Surgical incision should never be through the scrotal skin as this carries a risk of tumour contamination and this approach will not achieve adequate excision of the cord. The testis should be removed through an inguinal excision following high ligation of the cord. In children these tumours are normally predominantly of yolk sac elements and therefore produce AFP. When elevated it can be used as a useful diagnostic marker (Coppack et al., 1983) and only hepatoblastoma produces comparable levels of alpha-fetoprotein. Routine staging investigations should include chest X-ray/CT scan of chest and abdomen and bone scan.

If there is no evidence of metastatic disease surgical excision is likely to be curative. AFP levels should be followed weekly until normal and provided the elimination half-life is not prolonged (normally less than 5–7 days) no further action is required (Peckham et al., 1982). A slow half-life or a failure to reach normal levels necessitates further re-evaluation to seek persistent or recurring disease. An alternative marker is β-HCG which is elevated if there is a trophoblastic element. The half-life of HCG is 2–3 days. In remission, the patient should be followed with monthly AFPs for 12 months and then three monthly to two years, beyond which time the risk of relapse is minimal.

If the tumour does not produce AFP, a similar approach may be followed but with even closer clinical and ultrasound follow-up. In the event of relapse these patients are highly curable with chemotherapy.

Ovarian tumours

These present as an abdominal or pelvic mass often with abdominal pain (Figure 9.34). Occasionally there may be vaginal bleeding or amenorrhoea. Dysgerminomas or yolk sac tumours are the commonest histological types and up to 15% will be bilateral at presentation. Staging investigations are as for testicular tumours and with localized disease, unilateral salpingo-oophorectomy without postoperative radiation or chemotherapy will be curative in the majority of patients (Flamant *et al.*, 1978; Flamant *et al.*, 1984). With more extensive disease, chemotherapy is usually the primary treatment modality, to avoid the need for extensive mutilating surgery. This is a highly chemosensitive tumour and can be cured by chemotherapy alone (La Vecchia, Morris and Draper, 1983; Mann *et al.*, 1989; Pinkerton *et al.*, 1990).

Sacrococcygeal teratomas

These present in the neonatal period and usually have benign, well-differentiated pathology. Complete resection including excision of the coccyx is curative in the majority of cases. In some, usually those with extensive intra-abdominal disease or the older child, the pathology

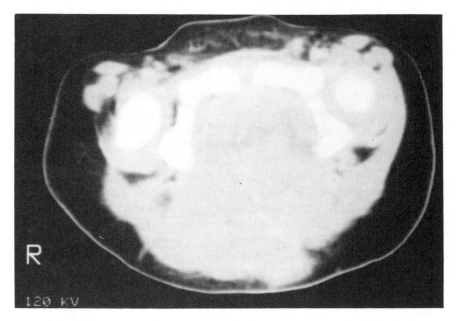

Figure 9.34 Very extensive sacrococcygeal tumour arising in an infant. The tumour completely fills the pelvis extending into the soft tissue at the base of the spine.

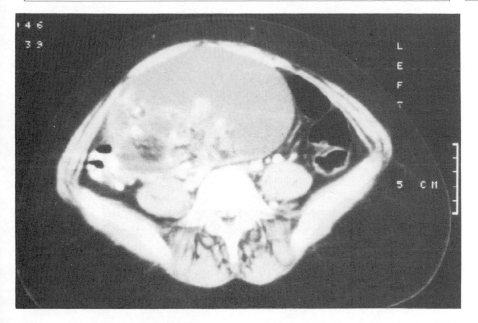

Figure 9.35 A right-sided ovarian teratoma. The heterogeneous pattern on CT reflects the mixed pattern of tissue differentiation in this mature teratoma.

may be more malignant with yolk sac or undifferentiated teratomatous elements. In late presentations there may be dysuria, difficulty with defaecation or neurological symptoms (Figure 9.35). Chemotherapy is very effective and the overall prognosis is good without the need for radiotherapy.

Mediastinal germ cell tumours

These are of mixed histological type and because they are often of great bulk at presentation may be particularly difficult to treat. With effective chemotherapy, however, followed by resection of any residual tumour, at least 50% should be cured (Logothetis *et al.*, 1985) (Figure 9.36).

High dose cyclophosphamide, doxorubicin, vincristine (CAV) is active in malignant germ cell tumours, but cisplatin or carboplatin, etoposide, bleomycin regimens are shorter, non-sterilizing and at least as effective (Flamant *et al.*, 1984; Mann *et al.*, 1989; Pinkerton *et al.*, 1990; Peckham *et al.*, 1983). The rate of decline of tumour marker or the time to complete radiological remission is taken as a guide to the duration of chemotherapy. Short courses of around six months are usually sufficient.

Residual masses after chemotherapy often consist of benign teratoma and should be resected if possible.

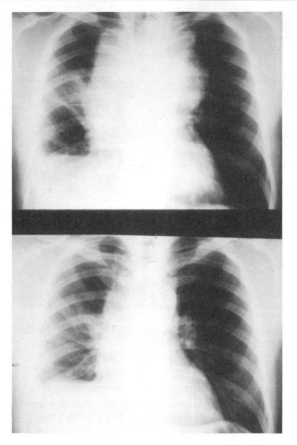

Figure 9.36 Mediastinal malignant germ cell tumour before and after chemotherapy with a cisplatin/etoposide based protocol.

REFERENCES

Leukaemia, lymphomas

Alexander, F.E. (1993) Viruses, clusters and clustering of childhood leukemia. A new perspective? *European Journal of Cancer*, **29A**, 1424–1443.

Behrendt, H., Van Bunningen, B.N.F.M. and Van Leeuwen, E.F. (1987) Treatment of Hodgkin's disease in children with or without radiotherapy. *Cancer*, **59**, 1870–1873.

Bennett, J.M., Catovsky, D. and Daniel, M-T. (1976) Proposals for the classification of the acute leukaemias. French-American-British (FAB) Co-operative Group. *British Journal of Haematology*, **33**, 451.

Bordigoni, P., Vernant, J.P., Souillet, E. *et al.* (1989) Allogeneic bone marrow transplantation for children with acute lymphoblastic leukemia in first remission:

A cooperative study of the Group d'Etude de la Greffe de Moelle Osseuse. *Journal of Clinical Oncology*, **7**(6), 747–753.

Brochstein, J.A., Kernan, N.A., Groshen, S. *et al.*, (1987) Allogeneic bone marrow transplantation after hyperfractionated total-body irradiation and cyclophosphamide in children with acute leukaemia. *New England Journal of Medicine*, **317**, 1618–1624.

Chessells, J.M. (1985) Cranial irradiation in childhood acute lymphoblastic leukaemia: time for reappraisal? *British Medical Journal*, **291**, 686.

Chessells, J.M., O'Callaghan, U. and Hardisty, R.M. (1986) Acute myeloid leukaemia in childhood: clinical features and prognosis. *British Journal of Haematology*, **63**, 555–564.

Craft, A.W., Openshaw, S. and Birch, J. (1984) Apparent clusters of childhood lymphoid malignancy in northern England. *Lancet*, **ii**, 96–97.

Donaldson, S.S. (1984) Editorial: Is involved field irradiation alone optimal therapy for a child with Hodgkin's disease? *Medical and Pediatric Oncology*, **12**, 322–324.

Editorial (1990) Childhood leukaemia: an infectious disease? *Lancet*, **336**, 1477–1478.

Ekert, H., Waters, K.D., Smith, P.J. *et al.* (1988) Treatment with MOPP or ChlVPP chemotherapy only for all stages of childhood Hodgkin's disease. *Journal of Clinical Oncology*, **6**, 1845–1850.

Gale, R.P. and Champlin, R.E. (1986) Bone marrow transplantation in acute leukaemia. *Clinics in Haematology*, **15**, 851–872.

Gardner, M.J., Snee, M.P., Hall, A.J. *et al.* (1990) Results of case-control study of leukaemia and lymphoma among young people near Sellafield nuclear plant in West Cumbria. *British Medical Journal*, **300**, 423–429.

Greaves, M.F. and Chan, L.C. (1986) Is spontaneous mutation the major 'cause' of childhood acute lymphoblastic leukaemia? *British Journal of Haematology*, **64**, 1–13.

Green, D.M., Choorah, J., Douglass, H.O. *et al.* (1983) Staging laparotomy with splenectomy in children and adolescents with Hodgkin's disease. *Cancer Treatment Reviews*, **10**, 23–28.

Jaffe, E.S. (1989) The elusive Reed–Sternberg cell. *New England Journal of Medicine*, **320**, 529–531.

Jenkin, D., Chan, H., Freedman, M. *et al.* (1982) Hodgkin's disease in children: Treatment results with MOPP and low-dose, extended field irradiation. *Cancer Treatment Reports*, **66**(4), 949–959.

Kjeldsberg, C.R. and Wilson, J.F. (1986) Malignant Lymphoma in Children, in *Pathology of Neoplasia in Children and Adolescents* (ed. M. Finegold), W.B. Saunders. Philadelphia.

Linch, O.C. and Burnett, A.K. (1986) Clinical studies of ABMT in acute myeloid leukaemia. *Clinics in Haematology*, **15**, 167–186.

Mueller, N.E. (1987) The epidemiology of Hodgkin's disease, in *Hodgkin's Disease* (eds P. Selby and T.J. McElwain), Blackwell, Oxford.

Patte, C., Philip, T., Rodary, C. *et al.* (1986) Improved survival rate in children with stage III and IV B-cell non-Hodgkin's lymphoma and leukemia using multiagent chemotherapy: Results of a study of 114 children from the French Pediatric Oncology Society. *Journal of Clinical Oncology*, **4**(8), 1219–1226.

Philip, T., Pinkerton, R., Biron, P. *et al.* (1987) Effective multiagent chemotherapy in children with advanced B cell lymphoma: who remains the high risk patient? *British Journal of Haematology*, **65**, 159–164.

Pinkerton, C.R., Bowman, A., Holtzel, H. *et al.* (1987) Intensive consolidation chemotherapy for acute lymphoblastic leukaemia (UKALL X pilot study). *Archives of Disease in Childhood*, **62**, 12–18.

Pinkerton, C.R. and Chessells, J.M. (1984) Failed central nervous system prophylaxis in children with acute lymphoblastic leukaemia: treatment and outcome. *British Journal of Haematology*, **57**, 553–561.

Reaman, G., Zeltzer, P., Bleyer, W.A. *et al.* (1985) Acute lymphoblastic leukemia in infants less than one year of age: a cumulative experience of the Children's Cancer Study Group. *Journal of Clinical Oncology*, **3**(11), 1512–1521.

Robinson, B., Kingston, J., Nogueira Costa, R. *et al.* (1984) Chemotherapy and irradiation in childhood Hodgkin's disease. *Archives of Disease in Childhood*, **59**, 1162–1167.

Russell, K.J., Donaldson, S.S., Cox, R.S. *et al.* (1984) Childhood Hodgkin's disease: patterns of relapse. *Journal of Clinical Oncology*, **2**, 80–87.

Sallan, S.E., Niemeyer, C.M., Billett, A.L. *et al.* (1989) Autologous bone marrow transplantation for acute lymphoblastic leukaemia. *Journal of Clinical Oncology*, **7**, 1594–1601.

Schroeder, H., Pinkerton, C.R. and Meller, S.T. (1991) High dose melphalan and total body irradiation with autologous marrow rescue in childhood acute lymphoblastic leukaemia. *Bone Marrow Transplantation*, **7**, 11–15.

Selby, P., McElwain, T.J. and Canellos, G. (1987) Chemotherapy for Hodgkin's disease, in *Hodgkin's Disease* (eds P. Selby and T.J. McElwain), Blackwell, Oxford.

Sieff, C.A., Chessells, J.M., Harvey, B.A.M. *et al.* (1981) Monosomy 7 in childhood: a myeloproliferative disorder. *British Journal of Haematology*, **49**, 235–249.

Tiedemann, K., Chessells, J.M. and Sandland, R.M. (1982) Isolated testicular relapse in boys with acute lymphoblastic leukaemia: treatment and outcome. *British Medical Journal*, **285**, 1614–1616.

Weiner, M., Leventhal, B. and Cantor, A. (1991) Gallium-67 scans as an adjunct to computed tomography scans for the assessment of a residual mediastinal mass in pediatric patients with Hodgkin's disease. *Cancer*, **68**, 2478–2480.

Wheeler, K. and Chessells, J.M. (1990) UKALL-X – an effective treatment for stage III mediastinal non-Hodgkin's lymphoma. *Archives of Disease in Childhood*, **65**, 252–254.

Brain tumours

Allen, J.C., Bloom, J., Ertell, I. *et al.* (1986) Brain tumours in children: current co-operative and institutional chemotherapy trials in newly diagnosed and recurrent disease. *Seminars in Oncology*, **13**, 110–122.

Allen, J.C., Kim, J.H. and Packer, R.J. (1987) Neoadjuvant chemotherapy for newly diagnosed germ cell tumors of the central nervous system. *Journal of Neurosurgery*, **67**, 65–70.

Bloom, H.J.G. (1982) Intracranial tumors: response and resistance to therapeutic endeavors, 1970–1980. *International Journal of Radiation Oncology Biology Physics*, **8**, 1083–1113.

Horwich, A. and Bloom, H.J.G. (1985) Optic gliomas; radiation therapy and prognosis. *International Journal of Radiation Oncology Biology Physics*, **11**, 1067–1079.

Johnson, D.B., Thompson, J.M., Corwin, J. *et al.* (1987) Prolongation of survival for high-grade malignant gliomas and adjuvant high-dose BCNU and autologous bone marrow transplantation. *Journal of Clinical Oncology*, **5**, 783–789.

Mananka, S., Teramoto, A. and Takakura, K. (1985) The efficacy of radiotherapy for craniopharyngioma. *Journal of Neurosurgery*, **62**, 648–656.

Packer, R.J., Sutton, L.N., Bilaniuk, L.T. *et al.* (1988) Treatment of chiasmatic/hypothalamic gliomas of childhood with chemotherapy: an update. *Annals of Neurology*, **23**, 79–85.

Pendergrass, T.W., Milstein, J.M., Geyer, J.R. *et al.* (1987) Eight drugs in one day chemotherapy for brain tumours: experience in 107 children and rationale for pre-radiotherapy chemotherapy. *Journal of Clinical Oncology*, **5**, 1221–1231.

Russell, D.R. and Rubinstein, L.J. (1977) *Pathology of Tumours of the Nervous System*, 4th edn, Williams & Wilkins, Baltimore.

Shalet, S.M., Gibson, B., Swindell, R. *et al.* (1987) Effect of spinal irradiation on growth. *Archives of Disease in Childhood*, **62**, 461–464.

Silverman, C.L., Palkes, H., Talent, B. *et al.* (1984) Late effects of radiotherapy on patients with cerebellar medulloblastoma. *Cancer*, **54**, 825–829.

Sposto, R., Ertel, I.J., Jenkin, R.D.T. *et al.* (1989) The effectiveness of chemotherapy for treatment of high-grade astrocytoma in children; results of a randomized trial. A report from the Children's Cancer Study Group. *Journal of Neuro-oncology*, **7**, 165–177.

Thomas, D.G.T., Anderson, R.E. and du Boulay, G.H. (1984) CT-guided stereotactic neurosurgery: experience in 24 cases with a new stereotactic system. *Journal of Neurology, Neurosurgery and Psychiatry*, **47**, 9–16.

Thomas, D.G.T., Davis, C.H., Ingram, S. *et al.* (1986) Stereotaxic biopsy of the brain under MR imaging control. *American Journal of Neurological Research*, **7**(1), 161–163.

Walker, R.W. and Allen, J.C. (1988) Cisplatin in the treatment of recurrent childhood primary brain tumors. *Journal of Clinical Oncology*, **6**, 62–66.

Wolff, S.N., Phillips, G.L. and Herzig, G.P. (1987) High-dose carmustine with autologous bone marrow transplantation for the adjuvant treatment of high-grade gliomas of the central nervous system. *Cancer Treatment Reports*, **71**, 183–185.

Woo, S.Y., Donaldson, S.S. and Cox, R.S. (1988) Astrocytoma in children: 14 years' experience at Stanford University Medical Center. *Journal of Clinical Oncology*, **6**, 1001–1007.

Neuroblastoma

Bourhis, J., Hartmann, O., Benard, J. *et al.* (1989) Relapse from a stage IV-S neuroblastoma and N-myc amplification. *European Journal of Cancer Clinical Oncology*, **25**, 1653–1655.

Brodeur, G.M., Seeger, R.C., Barrett, A. *et al.* (1988) International criteria for diagnosis, staging and response to treatment in patients with neuroblastoma. *Journal of Clinical Oncology*, **6**, 1874–1881.

Evans, A.E., D'Angio, G.J., Propert, K. *et al.* (1987) Prognostic factors in neuroblastoma. *Cancer*, **59**, 1853–1859.

Kemshead, J.T. and Pritchard, J. (1984) Neuroblastoma: Recent developments and current challenges. *Cancer Surveys*, **3**, 691–708.

Kretschmar, C.S., Frantz, C.N., Rosen, E.M. *et al.* (1984) Improved prognosis for infants with stage IV neuroblastoma. *Journal of Clinical Oncology*, **2**, 799–803.

Lewis, I., Lashford, L.S., Fielding, S. *et al.* (1991) A phase I/II study of [131]I mIBG in chemoresistant neuroblastoma. *Advances in Neuroblastoma Research*, **3**, 463–469.

Look, A.T., Hayes, F.A., Shuster, J. *et al.* (1991) Clinical relevance of tumor cell ploidy and N-myc gene amplification in childhood neuroblastoma: A pediatric oncology group study. *Journal of Clinical Oncology*, **9**, 581–591.

Matthay, K.K., Sather, H.N., Seeger, R.C. *et al.* (1989) Excellent outcome of stage II neuroblastoma is independent of residual disease and radiation therapy. *Journal of Clinical Oncology*, **7**, 236–244.

Moss, T.J., Reynolds, P., Sather, H.N. *et al.* (1991) Prognostic value of immunocytologic detection of bone marrow metastases in neuroblastoma. *New England Journal of Medicine*, **324**, 219–226.

Murphy, S.B., Cohn, S.L., Craft, A.W. *et al.* (1991) Do children benefit from mass screening for neuroblastoma? *Lancet*, **337**, 344–346.

Philip, T., Bernard, J.M., Zucker, R. *et al.* (1987) High dose chemoradiotherapy with bone marrow transplantation as consolidation treatment in neuroblastoma: an unselected group of stage IV patients over 1 year of age. *Journal of Clinical Oncology*, **5**, 266–271.

Pritchard, J., Germond, S., Jones, D. *et al.* (1986) Is high dose melphalan of value in treatment of advanced neuroblastoma? *Proceedings of the American Society of Clinical Oncologists*, **5**: A805.

Pritchard, J., Kiely, E., Rogers, D.W. *et al.* (1987) Long-term survival after advanced neuroblastoma. *New England Journal of Medicine*, **617**, 1026.

Shuster, J.J., Cantor, A.B., McWilliams, N. *et al.* (1991) The prognostic significance of autologous bone marrow transplant in advanced neuroblastoma. *Journal of Clinical Oncology*, **6**, 1045–1049.

Suarez, A., Hartmann, O., Vassal, G. *et al.* (1991) Treatment of stage IV-S neuroblastoma: A study of 34 cases treated between 1982 and 1987. *Medical and Pediatric Oncology*, **19**, 473–477.

Wilson, P.C.G., Coppes, M.J., Solh, H. *et al.* (1991) Neuroblastoma stage IV-S: A heterogeneous disease. *Medical and Pediatric Oncology*, **19**, 467–472.

Wilms' tumour

Azouz, E.M., Larson, E.J., Patel, J. *et al.* (1990) Beckwith–Wiedemann syndrome: development of nephroblastoma during the surveillance period. *Pediatric Radiology*, **20**, 550–552.

Berry, P.J. and Vujanic, G.M. (1992) Malignant rhabdoid tumour. *Histopathology*, **20**, 189–193.

Coppes, M.J., deKraker, J., van Dijken, P.J. et al. (1989) Bilateral Wilms' tumor: Long-term survival and some epidemiological features. *Journal of Clinical Oncology*, **7**(3), 310–315.

D'Angio, G.J., Breslow, N., Beckwith, B. et al. (1989) Treatment of Wilms' tumor. Results of the Third National Wilms' Tumor Study. *Cancer*, **64**, 349–360.

DeKraker, J., Lemerle, J., Voute, P.A. et al. (1990) Wilms' tumor with pulmonary metastases at diagnosis: The significance of primary chemotherapy. *Journal of Clinical Oncology*, **8**, 1187–1190.

Drash, A., Sherman, F., Hartmann, W.H. et al. (1970) A syndrome of pseudo-hermaphroditism, Wilms' tumor, hypertension, and degenerative renal disease. *Journal of Pediatrics*, **76**, 585–593.

Green, D.M., Fernbach, D.J., Norkool, P. et al. (1991) The treatment of Wilms' tumor patients with pulmonary metastases detected only with computed tomography: A report from the National Wilms' Tumor Study. *Journal of Clinical Oncology*, **9**, 1776–1781.

Lemerle, J., Voute, P.A., Tournade, M.F. et al. (1983) Effectiveness of preoperative chemotherapy in Wilms' tumor: results of an International Society of Paediatric Oncology (SIOP) clinical trial. *Journal of Clinical Oncology*, **1**, 604.

Marsden, H.B., Lawler, W. and Kumar, P.M. (1978) Bone metastasizing renal tumor of childhood. *Cancer*, **42**, 1922–1928.

Steinfeld, A.D., Crowley, C.A., O'Shea, P.A. et al. (1984) Recurrent and metastatic mesoblastic nephroma in infancy. *Journal of Clinical Oncology*, **2**(8), 956–960.

Weeks, D.A., Beckwith, J.B., Mierau, G.W. et al. (1989) Rhabdoid tumor of kidney. A report of 111 cases from the National Wilms' Tumor Study Pathology Center. *American Journal of Surgery and Pathology*, **13**(6), 439–458.

Soft tissue sarcomas

Crist, W.M., Garnsey, L., Beltangady, M.S. et al. (1990) Prognosis in children with rhabdomyosarcoma: A report of the Intergroup Rhabdomyosarcoma Studies I and II. *Journal of Clinical Oncology*, **8**, 443–452.

Flamant, F., Gerbaulet, A., Nihoul-Fekete, C. et al. (1990) Long-term sequelae of conservative treatment by surgery, brachytherapy, and chemotherapy for vulval and vaginal rhabdomyosarcoma in children. *Journal of Clinical Oncology*, **8**, 1847–1853.

Flamant, F., Rodary, C., Rey, A. et al. (1991) Assessing the benefit of primary chemotherapy in the treatment of rhabdomyosarcoma in children. Report from the International Society of Pediatric Oncology RMS 84 study. *Proceedings of the American Society of Clinical Oncologists*, **10**, Abstr. 1083.

Gasparini, M., Lombardi, F., Gianni, M.C. et al. (1990) Questionable role of CNS radioprophylaxis in the therapeutic management of childhood rhabdomyosarcoma with meningeal extension. *Journal of Clinical Oncology*, **8**, 1854–1857.

Gasparini, M. and Lombardi, F. (1986) Soft tissue sarcoma of children, in *Cancer in Children* (eds P.A. Voûte, A. Barrett, H.J.G. Bloom et al.), Springer-Verlag, Berlin, pp. 36–45.

Hamilton, C.R., Pinkerton, R. and Horwich, A. (1989) The management of paratesticular rhabdomyosarcoma. *Clinical Radiology*, **40**, 314–317.

Heyn, R., Ragab, A., Romey, B. et al. (1986) Late effects of therapy in orbital

rhabdomyosarcoma in children. A report from the Intergroup Rhabdomyosarcoma Study. *Cancer*, **57**, 1738–1743.

Horowitz, M.E., Pratt, C.B., Webber, B.L. *et al.* (1986) Therapy for childhood
soft-tissue sarcomas other than rhabdomyosarcoma: a review of 62 cases treated
at a single institution. *Journal of Clinical Oncology*, **4**, 559–564.

King, R.K. and Clatworthy, H.W. (1981) The pediatric patient with sarcoma.
Seminars in Oncology, **8(2)**, 215–221.

Kingston, J.E., McElwain, T.J. and Malpas, J.S. (1983) Childhood rhabdomyosarcoma: Experience of the Children's Solid Tumour Group. *British Journal of
Cancer*, **48**, 195–207.

Koscielniak, R.C., Flamant, F., Carli, M. *et al.* (1992) Metastatic rhabdomyosarcoma and histologically similar tumors in childhood: A retrospective European
multi-centre analysis. *Medical and Pediatric Oncology*, **20**, 209–214.

Lawrence, W. Jr, Gehan, E.A., Hays, D.M. *et al.* (1987) Prognostic Significance
of Staging Factors of the UICC Staging System in Childhood Rhabdomyosarcoma: A Report from the Intergroup Rhabdomyosarcoma Study (IRS-II)
Journal of Clinical Oncology, **5**, 46–54.

Maurer, H.M., Beltangady, M., Gehan, E.A. *et al.* (1988) The Intergroup Rhabdomyosarcoma Study – I: A final report. *Cancer*, **61**, 209–220.

Miser, J.S., Kinsella, T.J., Triche, T.J. *et al.* (1987) Ifosfamide with Mesna
uroprotection and etoposide: an effective regimen in the treatment of recurrent
sarcomas and other tumors of children and young adults. *Journal of Clinical
Oncology*, **5**, 1191–1198.

Newton, W.A., Soule, E.H., Hamoudi, A.B. *et al.* (1988) Histopathology of
childhood sarcomas. Intergroup Rhabdomyosarcoma Studies I and II: Clinico-
pathologic correlation. *Journal of Clinical Oncology*, **6**, 67–75.

Olive, D., Flamant, F., Zucker, J.M. *et al.* (1984) Paraaortic lymphadenectomy is
not necessary in the treatment of localized paratesticular rhabdomyosarcoma.
Cancer, **54**, 1283–1287.

Phillips, M.B. and Pinkerton, C.R. (1992) Pilot study of a rapid etoposide–cisplatin
regimen in paediatric soft tissue sarcomas. *European Journal of Cancer*, **28**,
399–403.

Pinkerton, C.R., Groot-Loonen, J., Barrett, A. *et al.* (1991) Rapid VAC high
dose melphalan regimen, a novel chemotherapy approach in childhood soft
tissue sarcomas. *British Journal of Cancer*, **64**, 381–385.

Raney, R.B. Jr., Gehan, E.A., Hays, D.M. *et al.* (1990) Primary chemotherapy
with or without radiation therapy and/or surgery for children with localized
sarcoma of the bladder, prostate, vagina, uterus, and cervix. A comparison of
the results in Intergroup Rhabdomyosarcoma Studies I and II. *Cancer*, **66**,
2072–2081.

Raney, R.B. Jr., Hays, D.M., Lawrence, W.Jr. *et al.* (1978) Paratesticular
rhabdomyosarcomas in childhood. *Cancer*, **42**, 729–736.

Reboul-Marty, J., Quintana, E., Mosseri, V. *et al.* (1991) Prognostic factors of
alveolar rhabdomyosarcoma in childhood. An International Society of Pediatric
Oncology Study. *Cancer*, **68**, 493–498.

Rodary, C., Flamant, F. and Donaldson, S.S. (1989) (for the SIOP-IRS Committee). An attempt to use a common staging system in rhabdomyosarcoma: A
report of an International Workshop initiated by the International Society of

Pediatric Oncology (SIOP). *Medical and Pediatric Oncology*, **17**, 210–215.
Rodary, C., Gehan, E., Flamant, F. *et al.* (1991) Prognostic factors in 951 nonmetastatic rhabdomyosarcoma in children: A report from the International Rhabdomyosarcoma Workshop. *Medical and Pediatric Oncology*, **19**, 89–95.
Rousseau, P., Flamant, F., Quintana, E. *et al.* (1992) Primary chemotherapy in rhabdomyosarcomas and other malignant mesenchymal tumors of the orbit: Results of the International Society of Pediatric Oncology MMT 84 study. *Proceedings of the American Society of Clinical Oncologists*, **11**, 370.

Bone sarcomas

Burgert, E.O., Nesbit, M.E., Garnsey, L.A. *et al.* (1990) Multimodal therapy for the management of nonpelvic localized Ewing's sarcoma of bone: Intergroup Study IESS-II. *Journal of Clinical Oncology*, **8**, 1514–1524.
Eilber, F., Giuliano, A., Eckardt, J. *et al.* (1987) Adjuvant Chemotherapy for Osteosarcoma: A Randomized Prospective Trial. *Journal of Clinical Oncology*, **5**, 21–26.
Goorin, A.M., Perez-Atayde, A., Gebhardt, M. *et al.* (1987) Weekly high-dose methotrexate and doxorubicin for osteosarcoma: the Dana–Farber Institute/The Children's Hospital – study III. *Journal of Clinical Oncology*, **5**, 1178–1184.
Jaffe, N., Robertson, R., Ayala, A. *et al.* (1985) Comparison of intra-arterial cis-diamminedichloroplatinum II with high-dose methotrexate and citrovorum factor rescue in the treatment of primary osteosarcoma. *Journal of Clinical Oncology*, **3**, 1101–1104.
Jurgens, H., Exner, U., Gadner, H. *et al.* (1988a) Multidisciplinary treatment of primary Ewing's sarcoma of bone. A 6-year experience of a European Cooperative Trial. *Cancer*, **61**, 23–32.
Jurgens, H., Bier, V., Harms, D. *et al.* (1988b) Malignant peripheral neuroectodermal tumors. A retrospective analysis of 42 patients. *Cancer*, **61**, 349–357.
Kinsella, T.J., Triche, T.J., Dickman, P.S. *et al.* (1983) Extraskeletal Ewing's sarcoma: Results of combined modality treatment. *Journal of Clinical Oncology*, **1**(8), 489–495.
Link, M.P., Goorin, A.M., Miser, A.W. *et al.* (1986) The effect of adjuvant chemotherapy on relapse-free survival in patients with osteosarcoma of the extremity. *New England Journal of Medicine*, **314**, 1600–1606.
Look, A.T., Douglass E.C. and Meyer W.H. (1988) Clinical importance of near-diploid tumor stem lines in patients with osteosarcoma of an extremity. *New England Journal of Medicine*, **318**, 1567–1572.
MacVicar, A.D., Olliff, J.F.C., Pringle, J. *et al.* (1992) Ewing sarcoma: MR imaging of chemotherapy-induced changes with histologic correlation. *Radiology*, **184**, 859–864.
Rosen, G., Caparros, B., Huvos, A.G. *et al.* (1982) Preoperative chemotherapy for osteogenic sarcoma: Selection of postoperative adjuvant chemotherapy based on the response of the primary tumor to preoperative chemotherapy. *Cancer*, **49**, 1221–1230.
Rosenberg, S.A., Flye, M.W., Conkle, D. *et al.* (1979) Treatment of Osteogenic

Sarcoma. II. Aggressive resection of pulmonary metastases. *Cancer, Treatment Reports, Rep.* **63**(5), 753–756.

Liver tumours

Finn, J.P., Hall-Craggs, M.S.A., Dicks-Mireaux, C. *et al.* (1990) Primary malignant liver tumours in childhood: assessment of resectability with high-field MR and comparison with CT. *Paediatric Radiology*, **21**, 34–38.

Ortego, J.A., Ablin, A. Haas, J. *et al.* (1989) Successful surgical resectability of liver tumours following continuous infusion chemotherapy with adriamycin–cisplatin. *Medical Paediatric Oncology*, **17**, 277.

Siegel, M.D., Siegel, S.E., Isaacs, H. Jr *et al.* (1980) Primary therapeutic management of unresectable and metastatic hepatoblastoma in children, report of four cases. *Medical Paediatric Oncology*, **4**, 297.

Retinoblastoma

Harnett, A.N., Hungerford, J.L., Lambert, G. *et al.* (1987) Modern lateral external beam (lens sparing) radiotherapy for retinoblastoma. *Ophthalmic Paediatric Genetics*, **8**, 53–61.

Hungerford, J., Kingston, J. and Plowman, N. (1986) Tumours of the eye and orbit, in *Cancer in Children* (eds P.A. Voûte, A. Barrett, H.J.G. Bloom *et al.*), Springer-Verlag, Berlin, pp. 223–227.

Kingston, J.E., Hungerford, J.L. and Plowman, P.N. (1987) Chemotherapy in metastatic retinoblastoma. *Ophthalmic Paediatric Genetics*, **8**, 69–72.

Yandell, D.W., Campbell, T.A., Dayton, S.H. *et al.* (1989) Oncogenic point mutations in the human retinoblastoma gene: their application to genetic counseling. *New England Journal of Medicine*, **321**, 1689–1695.

Histiocytic disorders

Alvarado, C.S., Buchanan, G.R., Kim, T.H. *et al.* (1986) Use of VP-16-213 in the treatment of familial erythrophagocytic lymphohistiocytosis. *Cancer*, **57**, 1097–1100.

Broadbent, V. and Pritchard, J. (1985) Histiocytosis X – current controversies. *Archives of Disease in Childhood*, **60**, 605–607.

Chu, A., D'Angio, D.J., Favara, B. *et al.* (1987) Histiocytosis syndromes in children. *Lancet*, **i**, 208–209.

Dungar, D., Broadbent, V., Yeoman, E. *et al.* (1989) The frequency and natural history of diabetes insipidus in children with Langerhans' cell histiocytosis. *New England Journal of Medicine*, **321**, 157–162.

Histiocyte Society Writing Group (1987) Histiocytosis syndromes in children. *Lancet*, **i**, 208–209.

McLelland, J., Broadbent, V., Yeomans, E. *et al.* (1990) Langerhans' cell histiocytosis: the case for conservative treatment. *Archives of Disease in Childhood*, **65**, 301–303.

Risdall, R.J., McKenna, R.W., Nesbit, M.E. *et al.* (1979) Virus-associated hemophagocytic syndrome. A benign histiocytic proliferation distinct from malignant histiocytosis. *Cancer*, **44**, 993–1002.

Tseng, A. Jr., Coleman, N., Cox, R.S. *et al.* (1984) The treatment of malignant histiocytosis. *Blood*, **64**(1), 48–53.

Germ cell tumours

Coppack, S., Newlands, E.S., Dent, J. *et al.* (1983) Problems of interpretation of serum concentrations of alpha-foetoprotein (AFP) in patients receiving cytotoxic chemotherapy for malignant germ cell tumours. *British Journal of Cancer*, **48**, 335–340.

Dehner, L.P. (1986) Gonadal and extragonadal germ cell neoplasms – teratomas in childhood, in *Pathology of Neoplasia in Children and Adolescents* (ed. J.L. Bennington), Saunders, Philadelphia.

Flamant, F., Caillou, B., Pejovic, M-H. *et al.* (1978) Prognostic factors in malignant germ cell tumors of the ovary in children excluding pure dysgerminoma. *European Journal of Cancer*, **14**, 901–906.

Flamant, F., Schwartz, L., Delons, E. *et al.* (1984) Nonseminomatous malignant germ cell tumors in children. Multidrug therapy in Stages III and IV. *Cancer*, **54**, 1687–1691.

La Vecchia, C., Morris, H.B., Draper, G.J. (1983) Malignant ovarian tumours in childhood in Britain, 1962–78. *British Journal of Cancer*, **48**, 363–374.

Logothetis, C.J., Samuels, M.L., Selig, D.E. *et al.* (1985) Chemotherapy of extragonadal germ cell tumors. *Journal of Clinical Oncology*, **3**, 316–325.

Mann, J.R., Pearson, A.D., Barrett, A. *et al.* (1989) Results of the United Kingdom Children's Cancer Study Group's malignant germ cell tumor studies. *Cancer*, **63**, 1657–1667.

Peckham, M.J., Barrett, A., Husband, J.E. *et al.* (1982) Orchidectomy alone in testicular Stage I non-seminomatous germ-cell tumours, *Lancet*, **i**, 678–680.

Peckham, M.J., Barrett, A., Liew, K.H., Horwich, A., Robinson, B., Dobbs, H.J., McElwain, T.J., Hendry, W.F. (1983) The treatment of metastatic germ-cell testicular tumours with bleomycin, etoposide and cis-platin (BEP). *British Journal of Cancer*, **47**, 613–619.

Pinkerton, C.R., Broadbent, V., Horwich, A. *et al.* (1990) JEB – a carboplatin based regimen for malignant germ cell tumours in children. *British Journal of Cancer*, **62**, 257–262.

<table>
<tr><td>

10

</td><td>

Emergencies and
supportive care

</td></tr>
</table>

The wide range of acute complications, which may be either tumour or treatment related, emphasizes the need for experienced paediatric nursing and medical staff to be involved in the care of all children with cancer. Centralization of services is the only way to provide adequate access to blood transfusion facilities and the other subspecialties which are invariably required.

10.1 SUPERIOR VENA CAVAL (SVC) OBSTRUCTION

Any tumour occupying the upper mediastinum is capable of compressing the vena cava and this is often associated with pressure on the lower trachea or upper bronchi. By far the commonest cause of SVC obstruction is T-cell non-Hodgkin's lymphoma but this may also occur with neuroblastoma, Ewing's sarcoma and Hodgkin's disease. Common symptoms are dyspnoea, particularly when lying down, chest discomfort, hoarseness due to recurrent laryngeal nerve compression or dry cough. At late stages confusion and other neurological symptoms may develop. On examination there is an obvious fullness in the face, often with some degree of plethora and cyanosis and examination of the fundi may show venous dilatation. There is often engorgement of the veins of the upper chest wall.

The main importance of recognizing this syndrome is the absolute contraindication to any sedation or anaesthesia for diagnostic procedures. The airway in these patients is often in a very precarious state and even lying flat may precipitate respiratory obstruction. This is one of the rare cases where therapy has to be instituted without a pathological diagnosis. The chest X-ray is usually suggestive of T-cell lymphoma with typical anterior mediastinal widening and often pleural effusion. Treatment with vincristine and prednisolone will produce a rapid response in most cases and in the absence of this rapid response an alternative diagnosis should be considered. Once the initial acute episode has passed a tissue diagnosis may be sought. With T-cell NHL diagnostic bone marrow may be sufficient or tissue obtained by transbronchial biopsy or thoracotomy. Radiation therapy will produce a similarly rapid response but in general chemotherapy is the treatment of choice. With this type of bulky highly chemosensitive tumour precautions to avoid tumour lysis syndrome arc vital (see later).

10.2 UPPER AIRWAY OBSTRUCTION

Any large solid tumour occupying the thorax may produce respiratory embarrassment. Posterior mediastinal tumours include neuroblastoma, primitive neuroectodermal tumour, Ewing's sarcoma, rhabdomyosarcoma and malignant germ cell tumour. To exclude the latter an urgent serum alpha-fetoprotein and βHCG must be done, and urgent urinary catecholamine assay may be diagnostic in neuroblastoma. If these are negative then empirical chemotherapy such as IVA or VAC is generally started if it is felt a diagnostic biopsy would be too dangerous. Again after a few days an invasive biopsy may be done and it is unlikely that histological features will have changed sufficiently to confuse the diagnosis.

10.3 TUMOUR LYSIS SYNDROME

Any highly chemosensitive tumour when breaking down, either spontaneously or following commencement of chemotherapy may produce toxic breakdown products, in particular uric acid from the breakdown of nucleic acid and release of phosphate from tumour cells. This syndrome is most commonly seen with B-cell NHL, T-cell NHL or any high white cell count leukaemia. It has been reported, but is extremely rare, with other solid tumours. The main complications are due to a urate nephropathy leading to an exacerbation of the hyperkalaemia associated with potassium release from lysed tumour cells.

The management of such a situation is summarized below. The most important feature is sufficient prehydration and adequate metabolic evaluation of the patient prior to and during commencement of therapy.

Particularly high risk patients include high count ALL (B and T cell) and bulky B- or T-cell non-Hodgkin's lymphoma.

Pre-induction studies must include:

1. Renal ultrasound – to demonstrate renal parachymal infiltration or occasionally in NHL an obstructive element due to node pressure. Chest X-ray

2. Baseline urate
   urea, creatinine
   electrolytes
   Ca, PO_4, Mg
3. Blood pressure
4. ECG
5. Weight
6. Central venous line advisable both for fluid administration and central venous pressure monitoring

Monitoring during induction (all cases with WCC $>50 \times 10^9/l$) should include:

1. Accurate urine output and CVP (if possible)
2. Hourly blood pressure
3. b.d. weight
4. ECG rhythm looking for hyperK (T elevation; wide QT)
5. Electrolytes 6-hourly; Ca, PO_4, 12-hourly (6-hourly if WCC $>100 \times 10^9/l$)

Preventative measures

Allopurinol 10 mg/kg daily i.v./p.o. to reduce urate precipitation in the tubules should start at least 12 hours prechemotherapy. Vigorous hyperhydration is essential and should also start at least 12-hours prechemotherapy.

At least $3 l/m^2/day$ of 4% dextrose 0.18% saline with no added KCl should be given and a good urine output ensured prior to chemotherapy – ≥3 ml/kg/hr. Frusemide may be used to achieve this having checked that fluid intake is adequate. Hydration should be calculated in addition to other losses, e.g. drains or nasogastric tube. Postoperative patients must have had all fluid loss made up before chemotherapy. It is vital that such patients have had adequate i.v. fluids preoperatively, while fasting for anaesthesia.

Other additives, e.g. Ca, are given as *clinically* indicated during first 48 hours. Low NaCl content solutions should be used to reduce the risk of urate supersaturation associated with high urinary sodium. Calcium supplements should not be given if PO_4 ↑ as this will risk $CaPO_4$ deposition in tubules. The combination of ↓↓ Ca and ↑↑ PO_4 is an indication to dialyse.

Alkalination of urine is probably unnecessary if fluid input is adequate and carries the theoretical risk of increased PO_4 or xanthine precipitation in the tubules.

The main tumour lysis is usually evident 8–24 hours after induction therapy starts.

No aminoglycosides or vancomycin should be given during this period.

Intervention

Electrolyte derangements should be corrected as they occur.

HyperPO$_4$, or hyperK

Hydration should be increased to ~4 l/m^2/day and urine output maintained with frusemide (2 mg/kg) as necessary, i.e. if output drops below 3 ml/kg/hr.

HypoCa

Infuse Ca gluconate if symptomatic (1–2 ml/kg 10% sol) over 24 hr – but anticipate and avoid any increased PO$_4$.

With seizures Ca gluconate i.v. (5–10 ml 10% sol) is given. CaCl$_2$ should be avoided, as this may produce local vein toxicity and ulceration.

Severe hyperkalaemia

If the K$^+$ is >5.5 mmol/l calcium resonium A (0.3 g/kg 8-hourly orally or 1.5 g/kg daily rectally) should be commenced.

If the K$^+$ is >6.0 mmol/l an insulin and dextrose infusion is indicated – Insulin (0.1 unit/kg) in dextrose (3 g/unit of insulin) over 30 minutes intravenously (50% dextrose has 0.5 g dextrose per ml).

If the K$^+$ is >6.0 mmol/l despite the above measures, consider dialysis.

Plasma filtration may be a useful alternative to dialysis especially if fluid overload alone is the problem. This is performed through a radial/brachial arterial line with central venous return of blood.

Peritoneal dialysis (PD) is usually the first choice in the event of:
– uncontrollable K$^+$ increase >6 mEq/l
                  PO$_4$ increase >4 mmol/l especially with symptomatic hypocalcaemia
– severe oliguria/anuria
– fluid overload, particularly if there is a large blood product input
– creatinine >1000 μmol/l, urea >50 mmol/l

In patients where there is massive renal infiltration at presentation with evidence of dysfunction, elective PD prior to induction chemotherapy may be justified and will enable the administration of hyperhydration with confidence. Low dose irradiation of infiltrated kidneys may improve function, but this is rarely used.

– Haemodialysis is used if there is contraindication to PD such as peritonitis or severe enterocolitis.

The most important factor in the management of high risk patients is anticipation of problems, accurate fluid balance monitoring and prompt early intervention.

10.4 TUMOUR-RELATED HYPERCALCAEMIA

Although this is a relatively common complication in adult oncology, it is only occasionally seen in paediatric practice. It is generally associated with disseminated malignancies such as alveolar rhabdomyosarcoma; it has also been reported with acute lymphoblastic leukaemia and non-Hodgkin's lymphoma, in addition to Ewing's sarcoma and neuroblastoma. The patient may have the classic symptoms of hypercalcaemia, such as gastrointestinal upset with nausea, vomiting, polyuria which may in some cases lead to dehydration (Leblanc *et al.*, 1984). Management consists initially of hyperhydration using normal saline with the addition of frusemide. Although steroids and calcitonin may have some transient effect, the most effective method of reducing hypercalcaemia is intravenous aminohydroxypropylidene biphosphonate (APD). An intravenous dose ($30\,\mathrm{mg/m^2}$) given over 8 hours produces a steady decline in serum calcium over the following 24–48 hours (Morton *et al.*, 1988). Ectopic prostaglandin E has also been implicated in some tumours and prostaglandin inhibitory drugs such as indomethacin have therefore been used.

One importance in recognizing hypercalcaemia at presentation is that modification of initial therapy may be required. It is inadvisable to give any potentially nephrotoxic drugs such as cisplatin or ifosfamide in this situation and alternative agents should be given depending on the tumour type.

10.5 SPINAL CORD COMPRESSION

Tumours associated with either an extradural metastatic deposit or extension of primary tumour into the spinal canal include neuroblastoma, Ewing's sarcoma and non-Hodgkin's lymphoma. Primitive neuroectodermal tumours and rhabdomyosarcomas may also present in this way (Figure 10.1).

The management of an individual patient will depend on age and likely diagnosis. There may be clear circumstantial evidence of the type of tumour, e.g. chest X-ray may show a paraspinal mass consistent with thoracic neuroblastoma or ultrasound may show an abdominal tumour. Both of these investigations can be done rapidly, although an emergency CT or MRI scan is advisable if possible. An urgent urinary catecholamine

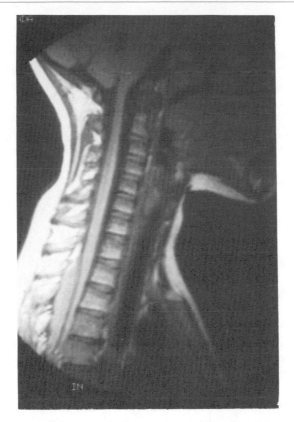

Figure 10.1 Acute spinal cord compression due to a plaque of extradural neuroblastoma causing thinning of the cord in the upper thoracic region.

assay may provide a diagnosis. Bone marrow aspirate may be diagnostic, and should be done particularly if there is evidence of myelosuppression. This could enable immediate institution of chemotherapy in the case of lymphoma or neuroblastoma. Although surgical decompression may appear to be the invariable treatment of choice, the late sequelae of multiple level laminectomy means that if possible this should be avoided. Lymphoma will be acutely chemo- or radiosensitive and there are many reports of a rapid response to chemotherapy alone in neuroblastoma and Ewing's sarcoma (Hayes *et al.*, 1981). The duration of neurological signs is also taken into account in making a decision about surgical decompression, as if these have been present for several days then the neurosurgeon may be more reluctant to operate. In the older child where the diagnosis cannot be obtained by non-invasive methods, then neurosurgery remains the treatment of choice.

10.6 SEIZURES

Generalized seizures may occur as a result of a primary brain tumour, or less commonly central nervous system leukaemia or lymphoma. More often it is associated with drug therapy such as busulfan, high-dose methotrexate, high-dose cytarabine or ifosfamide. Following bone marrow transplant cyclosporin A may lead to seizures, particularly when associated with hypertension and the use of high-dose methylprednisolone for graft versus host disease. Secondary metabolic dysfunction, for example hyponatraemia due to inappropriate ADH associated with vincristine may also lead to generalized fits.

10.7 ACUTE HAEMORRHAGE

Common causes and manifestations of bleeding are listed in Table 10.1. This is a problem either at the time of diagnosis in acute leukaemia, particularly the hypergranular promyelocytic form of AML, or during the period of profound myelohypoplasia following intensive pulsed chemotherapy, particularly where there is associated infection. Investigations and outline of management of acute haemorrhage are shown in Table 10.2. The tendency to use platelets prophylactically has recently lost favour and a much more conservative approach is generally applied (Table 10.3). Not only are platelets expensive but there is the risk of developing antiplatelet antibodies so that when the platelets are really needed in the event of a haemorrhage a poor increment is achieved and they are less effective. Moreover, they carry a risk of transmitting cytomegalovirus unless specifically screened for this. In general, patients who are likely to receive a bone marrow transplant procedure, i.e. AML or high risk ALL, should receive CMV-negative blood products from the time of diagnosis, unless they are known to be CMV positive. For this reason all such patients should have their CMV serology tested at presentation. This is because of the high risk of reactivation of cytomegalovirus following the profound immunosuppression of very high dose chemotherapy and transplantation.

Platelet reactions may occur usually due to the concomitant transfusion of small number of white blood cells. This may be prevented by the elective administration of 'cover' in the form of Piriton and hydrocortisone intravenously prior to transfusion. Alternatively, a leucocyte filter may be used. In general, the latter is only instituted where a platelet reaction has occurred, i.e. rash, chills, fever, shortly after commencing the infusion.

Although pooled multiple donor platelet transfusions are generally used, if a poor increment is achieved, i.e. minimal increase one hour after platelet transfusion, then it may be worth trying HLA matched platelets.

Table 10.1 Causes of haemorrhage

1. Thrombocytopenia
   chemotherapy
   post-marrow transplant
   disease infiltration
2. Coagulopathy
   disseminated intravascular coagulation (DIC)
   vitamin K deficiency/liver dysfunction
   asparaginase
3. Intestinal mucosal ulceration
   chemotherapy
   neutropenic colitis
   steroid induced gastric ulcer
4. Hyperleucocytosis

Manifestations
   petechiae, spontaneous bruising
   epistaxis
   mucosal; peridontal bleeding
   haematemesis, melaena
   haemoptysis
   retinal haemorrhage
   haematuria
   cerebral haemorrhage

Table 10.2 Diagnosis and management of coagulation disturbances

	Clinical Settings	Clotting Tests	Management
DIC	Septicaemia, AML (3) Any leukaemia with WBC > 100 × 10^9/l Disseminated sarcoma	Increased PT, PTT Decreased platelet count and short survival of transfused platelets Reduced fibrinogen Elevated fibrin degradation products	Treatment of underlying problem ? Heparin, cryoprecipitate (VIII) Platelet and fresh frozen plasma transfusions
Vitamin K deficiency	Severe malnutrition or liver dysfunction	Increased PT, PTT Normal platelet count and fibrinogen	Vitamin K (1–5 mg orally or i.v.) Fresh frozen plasma
L-asparaginase-induced coagulopathy		Increased PT, PTT Reduced fibrinogen	Temporarily discontinue L-asparaginase Fresh frozen plasma

This involves finding a donor from whom a single donation of platelets can be obtained using haemopheresis. A third method of obtaining platelets and one which is most appropriate in the event of an acute severe haemorrhage is to use a family member. Usually an ABO matched

Table 10.3 Indications for platelet transfusions

Count $<50 \times 10^9/l$ if:
   any significant bleed
   major surgical procedure
Count $<20 \times 10^9/l$ if:
   febrile
   minor surgical procedure, e.g. L.P.
   petechiae or mucosal bleed
Count $<10 \times 10^9/l$:
   if unlikely to recover rapidly
   unless chronically low with no haemorrhage or petechiae, e.g. delayed
   BMT engraftment

Table 10.4 Blood products commonly used in supportive care and prophylaxis

Products	Dose
Platelets	5 units/m^2
Packed red cells	Desired rise Hb $\times$ 6 $\times$ weight (kg) = volume transfusion
Fresh frozen plasma (FFP)	20 ml/kg
Purified protein fraction (PPF)	20 ml/kg
Albumin (20%)	5–10 ml/kg
Zoster immune globulin	2–5 yrs – 250 mg
	5–10 yrs – 500 mg
	>10 yrs – 750 mg
Measles hyperimmune globulin	0.15 ml/kg i.m.

sibling or parent is pheresed and in this way fresh platelets which are likely to achieve a good increment may be obtained.

Doses of blood products commonly used are given in Table 10.4.

Hyperleucocytosis and coagulopathies

An acute cerebral syndrome may be due to sludging of venous blood in cerebral vessels associated with very high count ALL, i.e. WBC >2–300 $\times10^9/l$ or due to intracerebral haemorrhage associated with the combination of disseminated intravascular coagulation (DIC) and profound thrombocytopenia.

DIC is a particular problem in acute myeloid leukaemia of the M3 (hypergranular promyelocytic) and M5 (monocytic) types and in these patients meticulous attention must be paid to the pretreatment and induction coagulation studies. DIC may, however, complicate any leukaemia particularly if there is associated septicaemia.

With hyperleucocytic leukaemias of whatever origin overtransfusion to correct anaemia must be avoided. If the anaemia is profound, i.e. less than 5 g/dl, slow correction over 2–3 days is appropriate. Rapid full correction may increase the risk of thrombosis. The management of DIC is as with any other cause, i.e. replacement of deficient factors with fresh frozen plasma (FFP) 5–10 ml/kg. If there is a profound poorly corrected hypofibrinogenaemia replacement with Factor VIII cryoprecipitate (rich in fibrinogen) may be appropriate.

The role of heparin in established DIC is unclear and not generally used. An exceptional situation is the elective use of low dose heparin infusion in hypergranular promyelocytic myeloid leukaemia. In this condition heparin is started immediately after diagnosis (100 units/kg/day continuous infusion) and continued for the first several days of induction, until the marrow is clear. This approach is an attempt to prevent the development of severe DIC associated with the release of granule products from blast cells during chemotherapy. Adequate platelet support is of utmost importance and levels must be electively maintained above $50 \times 10^9/l$ during initial induction. This may mean more than one transfusion per day if necessary and close surveillance of platelet increments achieved with transfusion.

Plasmapheresis has been occasionally used to reduce the blast cell mass, but the risks in an ill unstable child are rarely justified by the often small and transient reduction achieved. Similarly, early cranial irradiation pre-induction has been recommended to reduce the risk of blast cell associated complications, but this is not widely used.

It is important to reduce tumour burden as rapidly but as safely as possible. Full dose induction chemotherapy is started as soon as the diagnosis is clear. If there is diagnostic delay, vincristine and prednisolone or daunorubicin alone may be given as initial treatment.

Although fractionated cyclophosphamide and delayed adriamycin are used in advanced B NHL, in high count ALL or AML the full dose regimen is followed unless there are specific contraindications. These may be upper airway obstruction where vomiting is to be avoided and therefore daunorubicin delayed to day 2 or 3, or in very small infants where vincristine and prednisolone may be followed at 12–24 hours by daunorubicin.

10.8 SEPTICAEMIC SHOCK

Untreated infection may result in the child being readmitted with an established septicaemia. The clinical signs are usually a fever, although this is not always the case. The child is generally unwell and may be clammy with poorly perfused peripheries; there may be hypotension.

These clinical signs are an indication for the immediate commencement of broad spectrum antibiotics, having taken blood cultures and instituted intravenous hydration. Initial resuscitation with fluids such as normal saline or Haemaccel, or in some cases reconstituted plasma, may be necessary to re-establish blood pressure. The fluid volume given should be 10 mg/kg immediately followed by a further 10 ml/kg over half an hour. Then 10 mg/kg of 0.45N saline in 5% dextrose over the next 4 hours. During that time detailed plasma electrolytes should be determined before deciding on further hydration fluids. In some patients gastro-intestinal toxicity may lead to diarrhoea and the consequent dehydration will compound the situation. Severe hyponatraemia or hypokalaemia may be found and require appropriate correction (Glauser et al., 1991).

In some cases shock may lead to under-perfusion of the kidneys and a reduction in urine output. Low dose dopamine may be appropriate under such circumstances and once any dehydration has been corrected urine output may be re-established using frusemide.

In severe cases hypotension and bacteraemic shock lead to low output cardiac failure and high dose dopamine is required. In this situation as with any acutely unwell child an appropriately stocked crash trolley should be available at the time of initial resuscitation in case of cardiac arrest (Cohen and Glauser, 1991).

10.9 INTERSTITIAL PNEUMONITIS

The term interstitial pneumonitis (IP) refers to a radiological pattern in which there is diffuse bilateral hazy shadowing, often most marked in the hilar regions. This is due to cellular infiltration and oedematous fluid in the interstitial spaces due to a variety of organisms, which are listed on p. 218. Although the X-ray pattern is often typical, this may be variable and almost any pattern of infiltration can be seen in these conditions and X-ray alone is often insufficient to exclude a diagnosis (Figure 10.2).

The commonest clinical setting for interstitial pneumonitis is the child with leukaemia on continuing chemotherapy. The prolonged immuno-suppressive effect of 6-mercaptopurine is directly responsible for a pre-disposition to *Pneumocystis carinii*. The child presents with a history of dry cough, tachypnoea and exertion on exercise. Clinical examination reveals little else, in particular on auscultation, but on chest X-ray there is often a dramatic abnormality. In the child with more advanced disease blood gases typically show a low CO_2 and low oxygen level reflecting a compensatory hyperventilation, rather than the high CO_2 seen with bacterial pneumonia (Hughes, 1987).

The clinical setting is the most important consideration in deciding the likely cause. The majority of children with leukaemia now receive

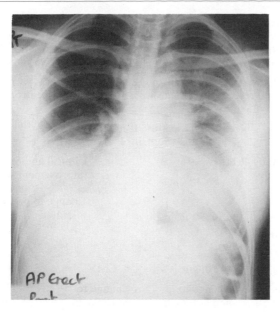

Figure 10.2 Bilateral pulmonary infiltrate associated with *Pneumocystis pneumoniae*.

prophylactic Septrin, given three times a week, which almost abolishes the risk of *Pneumocystis* (Enno *et al.*, 1978). Increasingly, however, the need to maintain chemotherapy doses during continuing treatment necessitates cessation of Septrin which can cause low blood count; inhaled pentamidine is an alternative approach (Golden *et al.*, 1989). *Mycoplasma pneumoniae* may be prevalent in the community and it is a likely pathogen, particularly in patients on Septrin. Fungal infections, such as *Candida* or aspergillosis generally result in more patchy or focal abnormalities on X-ray but in the profound immunosuppressed patient, for example following bone marrow transplant, this may not be the case. Respiratory syncytial virus may occur as part of a community outbreak. Radiation may be a contributory factor following total body irradiation or lung irradiation for lung metastases (Green *et al.*, 1989). Drugs responsible for a diffuse pulmonary infiltrate include bleomycin, high dose BCNU and, more rarely, methotrexate and high dose cyclophosphamide.

The approach to managing a child with diffuse pulmonary infiltrate is given in Table 10.5. Where possible a diagnosis should be made by bronchoalveolar lavage, so that treatment can be individualized. In general, however, high dose Septrin is combined with erythromycin in order to cover the two most common pathogens, namely *Pneumocystis* and *Mycoplasma* and erythromycin would also cover *Legionella*. The

Table 10.5 Management of diffuse pulmonary infiltrate

Bronchoalveolar lavage prior to treatment if feasible, but must not *delay* treatment in an unwell child

Initial treatment – May be individualized, e.g. BMT patient known to be CMV seropositive should receive early ganciclovir; ALL without neutropenia may have longer trial on Septrin

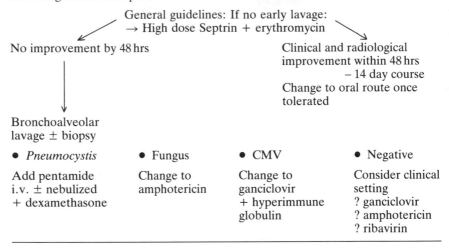

General guidelines: If no early lavage:
→ High dose Septrin + erythromycin

No improvement by 48 hrs

Clinical and radiological improvement within 48 hrs
– 14 day course
Change to oral route once tolerated

Bronchoalveolar lavage ± biopsy

• *Pneumocystis*	• Fungus	• CMV	• Negative
Add pentamide i.v. ± nebulized + dexamethasone	Change to amphotericin	Change to ganciclovir + hyperimmune globulin	Consider clinical setting ? ganciclovir ? amphotericin ? ribavirin

subsequent management will depend on the clinical picture as shown (MacFadden *et al.*, 1987; Browne *et al.*, 1990).

Decisions regarding the appropriateness of ventilating the child with cancer may be difficult, but again the overall clinical setting must be taken into account. Clearly in the child with leukaemia who is in remission on continuing chemotherapy and even in the face of severe *Pneumocystis* infection is likely to recover, there would be little hesitation in introducing ventilation. Conversely, the outcome in children with multiorgan failure following bone marrow transplant procedures is much poorer, but each case must be considered on its own merit. When introducing ventilation in the latter group, a clear strategy should be planned in advance and discussed at length with the family with regard to the likely duration of ventilation in the absence of any improvement. It is very distressing for the family to have a child on a ventilator for several days where no improvement is apparent. Clinical experience shows that in this situation recovery is very unlikely and it may be more humane to withdraw supportive care. The latter is, however, difficult once ventilation has been commenced.

10.10 ACUTE HYPERTENSION

The commonest types of hypertension in children with cancer the following:

Transient acute increase

- Postoperative
- Hypovolaemia with secondary hyper-reninaemia
- Hypocalcaemia
- Brain tumours or other CNS involvement
- Iatrogenic, i.e. fluid or blood product overload

Sustained hypertension

- Hyper-reninaemia associated with Wilms' tumour or less commonly neuroblastoma
- High catecholamines associated with neuroblastoma
- Obstructive uropathy with any abdominal or pelvic tumour
- Steroid administration, either iatrogenic or associated with rare adrenal tumours

Severe accelerated hypertension

This is hypertension where there is a risk of, or already established, secondary organ damage such as fundal changes, cardiac failure or neurological signs, such as visual loss or seizures.

Where it is directly tumour related chemotherapy may be the most appropriate therapy. In some settings, however, for example thrombocytopenia, there is some urgency in order to reduce the risk of cerebral haemorrhage.

Treatment approach (Table 10.6)

In the case of accelerated hypertension, labetalol infusion is generally the agent of first choice or, alternatively, nitroprusside. The latter may, however, have an adverse effect on platelet function. It should also be avoided if there is significant cardiomegaly and the addition of propranolol should be avoided. Sublingual nifedipine may also produce a rapid response but this can be short lived and more difficult to achieve sustained control. Therefore in general the above i.v. infusions are preferable.

Table 10.6 Management of hypertension

Exclude overhydration	Treatment: Lasix
	Reduce intake
Nifedipine	
– sublingual t.d.s.	
– slow release b.d.	
add hydralazine slow i.v. or p.o. b.d.	
+	
propranolol p.o. b.d.	

• Wilms'   • Neuroblastoma
   ↓   ↓
ACE inhibitor   Phenoxybenzamine p.o. b.d.
Captopril p.o. b.d.

Labetalol reserved for acute accelerated hypertension or severe unstable hypertension where intravenous route desirable

Moderate to severe hypertension

The agent of first choice is nifedipine and if the child is old enough to take a sustained release preparation this is probably preferable because of the more prolonged effect.

Second-line therapy is the addition of hydralazine and propranolol (N.B. contraindication to the use of propranolol in patients with asthma).

Third line can be disease orientated and in patients with a Wilms' tumour an ACE inhibitor such as captopril, which has a more effective antirenin effect can be added. In the case of neuroblastoma, specific α blockade with phenoxybenzamine is used. The strategy with refractory hypertension is to add rather than replace agents. Once control is achieved then the earlier used agents can be withdrawn. Nifedipine is kept for PRN use and hydralazine the first to be discontinued. Patients would, therefore, remain on propranolol plus either captopril or phenoxybenzamine.

Dose increase within each stage

In general doses should be increased in a three-stage process up to the maximum recommended dose. Generally one or two increases per day is appropriate.

Duration of antihypertensive therapy

This will depend on the cause. In the case of steroids, once medication is reduced or stopped the antihypertensives can be withdrawn. In neuroblastoma, if there is a response to chemotherapy withdrawal may be possible after a couple of weeks. In general this will be by trial and error with a gradual daily reduction in doses or elective removal of one drug in a multidrug combination.

Prophylactic antihypertensive cover in neuroblastoma

Because of the risk of surgically induced acute hypertension any child suspected of having a neuroblastoma on clinical grounds, who is going for a diagnostic biopsy, should be covered with phenoxybenzamine and propranolol for a 48-hour period starting 24 hours prior to surgery. If the patient has not been hypertensive preoperatively then these can be discontinued after 48 hours.

It is important that the blood pressure is related to age or height before a decision is made regarding the need to treat. In general, if it is above the 90th centile treatment is required.

10.11 INFECTION IN THE IMMUNOCOMPROMISED CHILD

The main barriers to infection in the healthy child are intact mucous membranes in the mouth and gastrointestinal tract; functional leucocytes and monocytes with an intact immune system capable of rapidly increasing the numbers of these cells in response to infection; functioning cell mediated immunity (CMI) capable of producing lymphocytes to deal with non-bacterial infections, and a functioning spleen to deal with specific infections such as *Pneumococcus*.

As splenectomy is no longer part of staging in Hodgkin's disease, loss of splenic function is a less common problem. However, following total body irradiation or extended field radiotherapy for Hodgkin's disease, there will be splenic dysfunction and prophylactic penicillin will therefore be necessary.

Mucosal ulceration is the consequence of many anticancer drugs, in particular the anthracyclines, actinomycin D, methotrexate and many forms of high dose therapy. Neutropenia *per se* may also induce oral ulceration.

The most important problem is, however, the neutropenia induced by chemotherapy. Few active drugs are devoid of significant myelo-suppression, the exceptions being asparaginase, vincristine and pred-nisolone. The timing of the nadir of the blood count varies with different drugs or combinations but generally is between 10 and 15 days following commencement of chemotherapy. Similarly, the duration of neutropenia will vary on the dose and number of drugs used. Although a neutrophil count of less than $1 \times 10^9/l$ is generally regarded as indicating a patient at significant risk, it has been shown that it is below a count of $0.2 \times 10^9/l$ that severe septicaemia tends to occur. In addition to neutropenia, both monocytopenia and lymphopenia will contribute to the predisposition to infection.

The poor nutritional status often associated either with the primary disease or with intensive chemotherapy also predisposes to infection.

The normal oral and intestinal flora is a delicate balance of organisms which competitively inhibit foreign organism growth, in particular that of *Candida*. Following intensive chemotherapy and broad-spectrum antibiotics floral patterns will change and this may lead to invasion by unusual bacteria or fungi.

Organisms commonly involved at individual sites of infection in myelosuppressed children:

1. *Septicaemia*
   Gram negative   *Pseudomonas*
     E. coli
     Klebsiella

   Gram positive   *Staph. aureus/epidermidis*
     Streptococcus
     Corynebacterium
     Listeria

   Anaerobes   *Bacteroides*
     Clostridium

2. *Lung*
   Bacterial   *Strep. pneumoniae*
     H. influenzae

     Klebsiella
     Pseudomonas
     Staph. aureus

   Viral   CMV, RSV

   Protozoal   *Pneumocystis*

   Fungal   *Candida*
     Aspergillosis

3. *Gastrointestinal tract*
   Oral mucosal   *Streptococcus*
   Periodontal   Anaerobes
     Candida

Oesophagus	*Candida*
	Herpes simplex
Intestinal	*Pseudomonas*
	Clostridium perfringens
	Clostridium septicum
	Clostridium difficile
	Campylobacter
	Giardia
Perianal	*Pseudomonas*
	Klebsiella
	E. coli
	Gp. D strep.

4. *Urinary tract*

    E. coli
    B. proteus
    Klebsiella
    Pseudomonas
    Enterococci

    Candida

5. *Cutaneous*

    Streptococcus/staphylococcus
    Pseudomonas
    Aspergillus/Candida/mucormycosis
    Herpes simplex/zoster

6. *Central nervous system*
  Meningitis

    Cryptococcus
    Listeria
    H. influenzae
    Neisseria meningitidis
    Meningococcus

  Brain abscess

    Staph. aureus
    Nocardia
    Aspergillus
    Candida
    Mucormycosis

  Encephalitis

    Herpes simplex
    varicella
    measles
    Toxoplasma

Table 10.7 Organisms commonly involved in neutropenic child and drugs to which they are usually sensitive

Infecting agent	Treatment options
Bacteria	
Pseudomonas	Piperacillin, Gentamicin, Ceftazidime, Ciprofloxacin
Klebsiella	Piperacillin, Gentamicin, Ceftazidime, Ciprofloxacin
E. coli	Piperacillin, Gentamicin, Ceftazidime, Ciprofloxacin
Staph. aureus	Flucloxacillin, Teicoplanin, Vancomycin, Cefuroxime
Staph. epidermidis	Vancomycin, Teicoplanin
Strep. pneumoniae	Penicillin V, Erythromycin
Meningococcus	Penicillin V, Chloramphenicol, Ceftazidime
Enterococcus	Ampicillin, Vancomycin, Ceftazidime
Bacteroides ⎱ *Clostridium* ⎰	Vancomycin, Metronidazole, Clindamycin
H. influenzae	Ampicillin, Septrin, Cefuroxime
Fungal/Protozoa	
Candida	Amphotericin/Ambisome, Fluconazole
Aspergillus	Amphotericin; Flucytosine; Itraconazole
Pneumocystis	High-dose Septrin; Pentamidine
Viral	
CMV	Ganciclovir; Foscarnet
Herpes simplex ⎱ Varicella/zoster ⎰	Acyclovir
R.S.V.	Ribovirin

Table 10.7 shows the drugs of choice for various organisms.

In the majority of cases if fever >38.5°C has been documented on two occasions 2 hours apart and the neutrophil count is $<1 \times 10^9/l$ treatment is started empirically before culture results are to hand. The initial investigations in this situation are as follows.

Initial investigations

A. Bacteriology

Blood cultures

Betadine in alcohol applied using a sterile gauze swab must be used for decontamination of patient's skin and individual bottle tops. The sampling needle must be discarded and a new needle used for the inoculation of each bottle.

Cultures must be taken from a peripheral site or through all lumens of the Hickman catheter (5–10 ml placed in each bottle). Two sets should be taken from each site. The interval between cultures is determined by the severity of the clinical condition. If bacterial endocarditis (SBE) is suspected 3 sets should be taken.

MSU
Sputum (if produced)
CSF (if indicated)

B. Virology

a. *Non-specific illness*
   Throat swab: in viral transport medium
   Urine: ×3 in viral transport medium (taken on consecutive days) for CMV isolation
   Stool: for virus isolation
   1st serum: 'PUO Acute Phase' (take second serum at 5–7 days)
b. *In acute respiratory tract infections*
   Sputum/nasopharyngeal aspirate:
   a. Viral immunofluorescence
   b. Viral isolation
   Throat swab and stool
   Sera: As above.
c. *Virology if vesicles present*:
   Vesicle fluid: On slide – for electron microscopy
   Swab of vesicle fluid: In viral transport medium for virus isolation
   Sera: As above.

C. Acute diarrhoea

Stool for: i.   Electron microscopy
             ii. Virus isolation
             iii. *C. difficile* toxin
             iv. Bacterial culture: including *C. difficile* and *Campylobacter*

D. Fungal infection

Blood cultures: Taken as previously but include Sabouraud's medium.

MSU and stool culture
Serum – for fungal serology

E. Chest X-ray and other imaging as indicated.

An antibiotic strategy is as follows and dosages for antibiotics in common use are shown in Table 10.8.

Table 10.8 Dosages for antibiotics, antifungal and antiviral drugs in common use in the paediatric unit

Drug	Route	Total daily dose (TDD)	Times daily (divide TDD by this fig)
Antibiotics			
Gentamicin	i.v.	6 mg/kg	3
Piperacillin	i.v.	300 mg/kg	4
Flucloxicillin	i.v.	50 mg/kg	4
Cefuroxime	i.v.	100 mg/kg	3
Ceftazidime	i.v.	100 mg/kg	3
Amikacin	i.v.	15 mg/kg	2
Metronidazole	i.v.	22.5 mg/kg	3
Chloramphenicol	i.v.	50–100 mg/kg (N.B. high dose for not longer than 48 hours)	4
Fucidin	i.v.	20 mg/kg	3
Vancomycin	i.v.	44 mg/kg	2
Imipenem	i.v.	25 mg/kg	6
Benzylpenicillin	i.v.	100 mg/kg	4
		300 mg/kg for severe infection	6
	i.t.	100 µg/kg	1
Ampicillin	i.v.	50 mg/kg	4
Erythromycin	i.v./p.o.	50 mg/kg	4
Ciprofloxacin	i.v.	10 mg/kg/day	2
	p.o.	15 mg/kg/day	2
Co-trimoxazole	i.v.	120 mg/kg (high dose for *Pneumocystis*)	4
	p.o.	Prophylaxis 240–960 mg	2
Teicoplanin	i.v.	12 mg/kg day 1 then 6 mg/kg daily	1
Antifungal			
Amphotericin	i.v.	0.25–1.0 mg/kg increase over 2 days	1
Fluconazole	i.v.	6 mg/kg – treatment	1
	p.o.	2 mg/kg – prophylaxis	
Antiviral			
Acyclovir	i.v.	15 mg/kg (*H. simplex*)	3
	i.v.	30 mg/kg (*H. zoster* and disseminated infections)	3
Acyclovir	Oral	*H. simplex* <2 yr 200 mg 2–10 yr 400 mg *H. zoster* <2 yr 400 mg >2 yr 800 mg	5 times/day

Fever in neutropenic child ($<1.0 \times 10^9/l$)

First line

Piperacillin; Gentamicin; Flucloxacillin.

Temperature settles
- culture positive
  treat for 7 days minimum
- culture negative
  stop once afebrile for 72 hr and neutrophils $>0.2 \times 10^9/l$

Temperature persists >48 hr
or clinically unwell >24 hr
  culture positive – treat accordingly
  culture negative – inflamed line – change flucloxacillin to vancomycin
    or empirical change to second line.

Second line

ciprofloxacin or ceftazidime; gentamicin; teicoplanin or vancomycin

Temperature persists further >48 hr
or clinically unwell >24 hr

Add amphotericin
- Acyclovir, if indicated, i.e. severe mucositis or vesicular lesions
- Metronidazole, if indicated, i.e. *C. difficile* toxin or major GI toxicity. *Not* just diarrhoea.

Line infection in non-neutropenic child

- Teicoplanin single agent $\times$ 5–7 days if outpatient
- Vancomycin if inpatient

The individual unit's policy regarding empirical treatment will depend upon the local flora and if particular organisms with particular sensitivity or resistance spectra are prevalent then this should be taken into account. Occasionally if the child is well and there are clear clinical signs of a viral infection, e.g. of the upper respiratory tract, a period of observation is appropriate, but in general there must be a very low threshold to start intravenous antibiotics. It is better to overtreat than undertreat such patients. As soon as blood culture results are obtained appropriate modifications should be made. In some units initial monotherapy with broad-spectrum agents such as ceftazidime or ciprofloxacin are used (Shenep *et al.*, 1988). This may be appropriate for patients who have received comparatively less intensive treatment regimens, such as for some solid tumours. However, any monotherapy regimen will result in a higher failure rate as no single drug provides complete cover against the spectrum of gram-negative and gram-positive organisms that may be involved. In the profoundly myelosuppressed or unwell child a delay to treat appropriately may be of grave consequence and for this reason monotherapy is in general not recommended.

The empirical change from one broad-spectrum antibacterial combination to a second one without support from blood cultures is debatable and in the well child with a comparatively high count there may be some flexibility. Of more importance is the strategy of introducing antifungal agents early which has had an important impact on morbidity and mortality in children with prolonged neutropenia (Cohen, 1982; Wiley *et al.*, 1990; Edwards, 1991).

Use of antifungals

Amphotericin

Start with test dose of 0.5 mg, then give 0.25 mg/kg over 4 hours. Increase to 1 mg/kg on second and subsequent days. In *proven* infection, escalate to 1.5 mg/kg. Alternate day administration can be used after day 3, i.e. doses on day 1, 2, 3, 5, 7 etc. Increasingly the liposomal bound amphotericin preparation Ambisome is being used (Chopra, Fielding and Goldstone, 1992); it is significantly less nephrotoxic and avoids the need for potassium replacement. A daily 1 hour infusion of 1–3 mg/kg is given. At present this preparation is suitable for empirical use but in established fungal infection amphotericin B should be used.

Discontinue once afebrile for 72 hr and neutrophils $>0.5 \times 10^9/l$ unless there is clear clinical or culture evidence of systemic/pulmonary infection when a prolonged course is required. The duration will depend on the speed of response, count etc.

If aspergillosis is present, treat with amphotericin. If slow response consider the addition of itraconazole, otherwise this agent is used as outpatient continuation treatment/prophylaxis in selected cases.

Fluconazole

This is given as a prophylactic in children who cannot take nystatin/fungizone in a dose of 1 mg/kg/d. For oropharyngeal *Candida* give 2 mg/kg/d and for systemic *Candida* give 6 mg/kg/d.

These guidelines show one strategy in which some patients may be relatively overtreated but at the end of the day the risk of overwhelming septicaemia or fungal infection is low. In the past donor granulocyte transfusions have been used but there are many arguments against their use, such as the potential risk of introducing CMV and the expense. Moreover, there are no randomized studies clearly showing benefit from this procedure.

With the increased use of indwelling central venous catheters, line infections have become a major problem. Although these are usually gram positive, e.g. *Staph. epidermidis*, gram-negative organisms may be implicated (see below).

Management of line infection in non-neutropenic child

First line antibiotic – vancomycin or teicoplanin.

If culture positive/temperature lowers then 7 days treatment.

If culture positive/temperature persists remove line and continue 24 hr antibiotic.

Flucloxacillin is rarely adequate as a single agent.

If blood culture grows a gram-negative organism, treat according to sensitivities but have a lower threshold to remove line if temperature fails to settle.

Persistent tunnel infection may necessitate line removal even if temperature lowers and culture is negative.

Bone marrow growth factors

In the last few years the structure of a number of naturally occurring haemopoietic growth factors has been determined and using molecular engineering have been synthesized. Examples of this are recombinant human GM-CSF (granulocyte monocyte colony stimulating factor) and G-CSF (granulocyte colony stimulating factor). These agents have the ability to stimulate the white cell count several fold when given to non-myelosuppressed patients. There is considerable interest in their role when given following intensive chemotherapy, in either preventing or shortening the period of neutropenia. Unfortunately the main drawback from these is that they have little, if any, effect on platelet count and moreover have to be given parenterally, either intravenously or subcutaneously over several days. Due to the considerable cost and inconvenience of the latter, it is essential that there is a clearly demonstrated beneficial effect in terms of reduced febrile neutropenic episodes, reduced duration of antibiotics and decreased hospital stay. Some studies in adults have suggested that this is the case but to date there are no clear studies in children showing their benefits. When given at the time of bone marrow recovery just following the nadir of white cell count, there is little doubt that count recovery will be accelerated and in this setting their use may be appropriate for treating patients who are admitted with febrile neutropenic episodes. There is some evidence that giving these factors during the early phase of profound myelosuppression, either post intensive chemotherapy or post bone marrow transplant procedures, is of benefit (Antman *et al.*, 1988; Brandt *et al.*, 1988; Metcalf, 1989). Increasingly G-CSF is used in the clinical setting where granulocytes were previously used as they may produce a rapid rise in neutrophil count within 48 hours and aid both tissue healing and resolution of fever.

Indications for bone marrow growth factors

In the presence of neutrophil count $<0.2 \times 10^9/l$:

1. Focal sepsis, e.g. severe cellulitis, not improving on antibiotics.
2. Culture-positive septicaemia, not responding to appropriate antibiotics.
3. Severe mucositis and intestinal toxicity.

Viral infections

Contact with other children with infections is a frequent source of anxiety. The periods of infectivity of the commoner diseases are shown in Table 10.9. Passive immunization with zoster immune globulin (ZIG) or pooled hyperimmune globulin (HIG) is recommended within 72 hours of contact (Table 10.4). Acyclovir should be used to treat any child with overt chickenpox or shingles. In general, viral infections, apart from measles and chickenpox will be uneventful, e.g. mumps and rubella. Routine immunization should be boosted six months after cessation of chemotherapy (full reimmunization after 12 months in the case of a marrow transplant).

Nutrition and the child with cancer

One out of every two children with cancer will exhibit symptoms of malnutrition at some stage (Donaldson, 1982). The child may present with nutritional problems as a result of their tumour or will develop a problem as a result of treatment (Woods, 1989).

Table 10.9 Periods of infectivity in childhood infectious diseases

Chickenpox	2 days before rash → 6 days after last crop
Measles	From onset of prodromal symptoms → 4 days after onset of rash
Mumps	3 days before salivary swelling → 7 days after
Rubella	7 days before onset of rash → 4 days after
Scarlet fever	10–21 days after onset of rash (shortened to 1 day by penicillin)
Whooping cough	7 days after exposure → 3 weeks after onset of symptoms (shortened to 7 days by antibiotics)

Children need good nutrition for their growth and development. This requires the provision of all essential food elements including protein, fat, carbohydrate, water, mineral salts and vitamins. Although several factors which will be detailed later may contribute to nutritional problems in the child with cancer, the basic problem is usually a lack of intake.

Donaldson (1982) defines malnutrition as inadequate growth with the weight:height ratio below the 20th percentile of the national standard. If weight loss is allowed to continue a state of cachexia will result. An individual's basal metabolic rate, that is the amount of energy required to provide the cells of the body with the necessary energy to carry out basic activities, determines the nutritional requirement that the individual needs. If they are not met energy reserves are used up in an attempt to make up the deficit. This process is gluconeogenesis, i.e. the formation of sugar (energy) from protein or fat where there is lack of available carbohydrate. If there is no intervention the result will be a wastage of lean muscle and adipose tissue, early satiety, lack of energy and increased weakness. Eventually there will be a decline in all motor activities leading to weakness in the respiratory muscle, thus a deterioration in the respiratory capacity leading to death. The latter is of course uncommon, but lesser degrees of malnutrition impair tissue healing, lead to poor tolerance of therapy and may result in suboptimal treatment.

Effects of treatments

Some diagnoses are associated with weight loss, e.g. advanced neuroblastoma, sarcoma or lymphoma, and require early active intervention. Such children are often with the poorest prognosis and are treated with the most aggressive therapies therefore compounding the problem of malnutrition. These therapies may be one, any combination of, or all of the following: surgery, chemotherapy and radiotherapy.

Surgery

The procedure itself will place great stress on the body, but more significant is the site and the extent of the surgery. Surgery to the head and neck may be radical and affect mastication or swallowing of food. This is rare however in childhood tumours, unlike adults, where preoperative chemotherapy usually avoids the need for debilitating surgery. Surgery to the gastrointestinal tract may result in the inability to eat for many days but in most cases is limited to biopsy only. Nutritional requirements will also increase in order to facilitate wound healing.

Chemotherapy

The side effects of cytotoxic drugs are many and the child may be lucky enough to experience none as regards potential nutritional problems, or experience many including anticipatory nausea and vomiting. Other side effects range from anorexia, mouth ulceration, infections, diarrhoea with subsequent fluid and electrolyte imbalance, to severe constipation resulting in gut stasis or ileus. Taste changes, decreased smell, abnormal taste are all potential side effects which may cause anorexia and subsequent weight loss (Trogdon Wall and Gabriel, 1983; Strohl, 1983).

Radiotherapy
Taste changes are an early complication associated with radiotherapy to the oropharynx. Xerostoma is very common in patients receiving radiotherapy to the head and neck and may be permanent in patients receiving high-dose radiotherapy (Westcott *et al.*, 1978). Radiotherapy to the abdomen and pelvis may result in diarrhoea with subsequent electrolyte imbalance. Radiotherapy to any part of the gastrointestinal tract may cause nausea and vomiting resulting in anorexia and weight loss (Donaldson, 1977).

Nutritional support
Successful management of nutritional problems is dependent upon practical solutions being made available to the patient's family. The family is the normal provider of the child's nutrition and the mother, in particular, usually feels that this aspect of her child's care is something she should be able to do something about. The treatment of cancer results in many unpleasant side effects which will alter the normal diet of the child.

Anorexia may be an isolated side effect of specific treatment, or may be secondary to many others, e.g. nausea, constipation. Being in hospital is traumatic and associated with much anxiety. Loss of appetite may be in response to unfamiliar surroundings, smells or different meal times and food. To overcome this problem, the family should be involved in their child's diet, choosing from the menu. The use of a ward kitchen at all times facilitates the ability to provide food at the child's normal meal times and to be able to provide food in smaller amounts more often if necessary. If the child's condition permits, encouraging cooking as part of occupational therapy may help. Nutrition can easily develop into an issue between child and mother and although it may be difficult for them to remain relaxed, the parents must be encouraged to do so and try to make the most of when the child does want to eat.

Taste change is often a side effect of chemotherapy or radiotherapy to the head and neck. There are approximately 10 000 taste buds on the tongue differentiating the sensations of sweet, sour, salty and bitter. During treatment for malignancies the cell turnover of the taste buds is altered and many children report that their food 'doesn't taste right'. In an extensive work on taste alterations in the patient with cancer DeWys and Walters (1975) report that there is a direct correlation between alteration in taste and weight loss; the patients who did not have weight loss were those who did not experience taste changes. Taste changes are partially restored 20–60 days after cessation of treatment and in most are completely restored at between 60–120 days. However, a small number of patients will have residual hypogeusia (Deweys, 1978).

Altered taste is not easy to overcome particularly if the child has another associated problem, e.g. mucositis. In such cases parenteral nutrition may have to be considered. With isolated taste loss practical ideas are dependent on the description of the taste experienced. Metallic tastes may be disguised with sharp or acidic flavours, e.g. lemon juice or vinegar. Salty taste may be lessened with sugar and vice versa. The child will need to experiment with foods and will often fancy something in particular and then discard it. Parents will become both frustrated and distressed by this and may interpret the situation as the child being difficult. Education of the family is of vital importance to explain that firstly this is normal and secondly that it is temporary.

Nausea and vomiting are very distressing and make temptation by food virtually impossible. Although worsened by smells (Guyton, 1976) nausea and vomiting are temporary. Many children receive short pulses of chemotherapy every few weeks and the emphasis on nutrition should occur between treatments, away from sights, sounds and smells of food associated with chemotherapy and hospitalization. For those children with prolonged admission when nausea and/or vomiting is a problem, parents should be advised to provide small amounts of food often with plenty of fluids in between. Strong aromatic foods should be avoided. It may be useful to allow the child to watch television at the same time so that the child is not aware of the prime focus of the exercise. For those children receiving emetic regimens regular anti-emetics will be given and those who may be experiencing delayed emesis, planned anti-emetics prior to meal times may be beneficial. A dietitian should be actively involved at all times with ideas to increase the calorie intake for when the child feels like eating. Where prolonged admissions result in substantial weight loss, alternative methods, for example, parenteral or enteral feeding, may need to be seriously considered.

Mucositis and ulceration result from inhibition of normal mucosal cell turnover due to either radiotherapy or chemotherapy and may lead to sloughing of the oral or oesophageal mucosa. Eating and swallowing becomes very difficult, unpleasant and often painful. Prevention, if possible, is desirable and can sometimes be achieved by regular mouth care regimens throughout treatment. Early intervention with acyclovir may be beneficial even in the absence of proven herpes infection. Similarly, systemic antifungal therapy such as low-dose amphotericin or fluconazole may avoid secondary candidal infection. If, despite rigorous mouth cleansing, sores do develop, local anaesthetic solutions such as xylocaine or

Difflam may make eating possible. However, severe mucositis often requires strong analgesia such as continuous infusion diamorphine, which should be started early rather than late. At times this will be enough to allow the child to eat a sloppy bland diet, but more often parenteral feeding will be considered.

Dry mouth or xerostomia due to the radiotherapy to the salivary glands results in reduced production of the saliva and the saliva produced is often thick and tacky. This occurs after either local irradiation or total body irradiation. The aim of treatment in such circumstances is to provide moist nutritious foods which are easy to swallow despite the lack of saliva. Frequent nutritious drinks should be offered to moisten the mouth. Sucking sweets helps to stimulate the salivary glands and any food offered should have plenty of gravy and sauce to aid swallowing. Artificial saliva may prove beneficial in some patients.

Diarrhoea which results when impaired absorption and increased mucosal fluid loss occurs due to the cytotoxic effects on epithelial cells of the intestinal tract. Fluid loss must be replaced; the volume may necessitate the intravenous route. Fluid balance becomes crucial as children have relatively higher percentage of body water than adults. A 5% loss of body fluid is a serious threat to a child's life and 15% loss can be fatal. Any food which may aggravate the condition should be avoided, i.e. those foods rich in fibre. Fluids such as Dioralyte which replace some of the mineral salts lost in the diarrhoea, may be prescribed if the child can tolerate this. After intensive chemotherapy the effect on the gastro-intestinal tract may be so severe that parenteral feeding is often necessary.

Constipation may be caused by the disease itself, treatment or from analgesia. Dietary advice is aimed at high fibre foods including wholemeal foods and fruit but equally important, plenty of fluids.

Developing an appropriate nutrition care plan will depend on the medical goals. If treatment is aggressive with an aim of a long remission or cure then the nutritional plan should also be aggressive (Lum and Gallagher-Allred, 1984). Regardless of the goals the dietitian, nursing staff and parents of the children must work closely together.

If the child is receiving palliative treatment or is already in the terminal stages of illness, the aims will be for comfort and enjoyment of life. The difficulty for the family to come to terms with this should not be under-estimated and many parents will ask for aggressive intervention for their dying child. The child should be allowed to eat whatever they like, whenever they like and in a comfortable relaxed atmosphere.

For the children receiving aggressive therapy and in whom weight loss is already a problem or is likely to become a problem, enteral (nasogastric or nasojejunal) or parenteral (total parenteral nutrition, TPN) nutrition are the treatments of choice in order to maintain the child in a good nutritional state.

Enteral nutrition using nasogastric or nasojejunal feeding tubes requires a functioning gut but is generally superior to TPN. For enteral feeding to succeed, the child needs to be able to tolerate the feed and therefore unless emesis is controlled during chemotherapy regimens, an alternative means of feeding needs to be considered. Also a child with mucositis will find the procedure very distressing. The advantage of enteral feeding is the ability to educate the parents in the administration of feeds to continue at home. Apart from the obvious benefit to the child, the parents will feel useful in actively participating in the well-being of their child.

Ready-made preparations for enteral feeding are commercially available and the aim is to provide proteins, vitamins and minerals to meet the patient's individual requirements (Table 10.10). The dietitian is responsible for calculating the calorie requirements and ensuring that the volume of fluid is realistic for the child to tolerate. The feed is introduced gradually and assessed each day in terms of tolerance, i.e. has the child developed diarrhoea or is vomiting a new problem? To allow the child to take part in normal childhood activities of schooling and socialization, the feed should ultimately be given overnight. Each child is assessed individually as to whether the nasogastric tube is left *in situ* or repassed every evening so that the child does not have another constant external reminder of his illness. Although most nutritional deficits are assessed and corrected during hospital admission this is not absolutely necessary. Once a care plan is decided and the child is tolerating the total volume of feed, assessment in terms of weight at each hospital visit will determine success.

Table 10.10 Nasogastric feeding preparations

	Daily intake	Energy/nitrogen (kJ/g)
Whole Protein		
Complan/Caloreen	280 g/200 g	840
Sobee	485 g	490
Sobee/Caloreen	260 g/215 g	840
Clinifeed 400	1980 ml	600
Clinifeed LLS	1650 ml	480
Hydrolysates		
Albumaid/Caloreen	75 g/450 g	840
Flexical	625 g	1500
Synthetic Amino Acids		
Aminutrin/Calonutrin	75 g/440 g	840
Vivonex	700 g	1120
Vivonex H.N.	575 g	530

Parenteral nutrition can be given irrespective of gut function. It has been suggested that any patient whose hospital stay is expected to exceed 15 days, who is unable to ingest, digest or absorb nutrients via the gastrointestinal tract is a potential candidate for intravenous nutritional support. The objective for parenteral nutrition is to provide adequate nutrients for the metabolic needs of the patient, replenish fat and muscle in malnourished patients and promote growth and development (Haas-Beckert, 1987). Long-term venous access needs to be available either via a Hickman catheter or a Portacath. The fluid administered is a combination of water, carbohydrates, fats, electrolytes, vitamins and minerals (Table 10.11).

Total parenteral nutrition is introduced over several days with a slow increase in the glucose content. By doing this the pancreas is able to adapt to the high glucose content that is necessary to provide adequate calories and increase the insulin output accordingly. Urinalysis and blood sugar levels are monitored.

The second major calorie source in TPN is fat in the form of lipids. These may adversely affect liver function and this must therefore be checked regularly. TPN may continue as long as necessary. Either the child's condition will improve enough to maintain nutritional intake, or the gastrointestinal tract is functioning again and the enteral means of feeding can be introduced. In some situations, TPN is required in the long term. This can be carried out at home, but only after considerable thought. Education of parents, a support system, is imperative with very frequent assessments.

The dietitian, nursing staff and parents of the children will not only be concerned with those children who present or develop nutritional problems. Many children will avoid significant weight loss due to the early detection of anorexia or slight weight loss leading to the introduction of a practical, effective care plan. In addition to advice given for specific problems, e.g. nausea, anorexia or constipation, there are many high calorie, high protein products available to boost the child's diet. Maxijul Supersoluble is a good example. This product is a tasteless glucose polymer with 4 calories per gram which can be added to drinks, gravies and sauces without the child being aware. There are also many high protein milky drinks which are now produced in many tempting flavours as well as flavoured glucose drinks.

In the past it was believed that undernourishment in the patient reduced the rate of tumour growth and therefore it was not unreasonable to conclude that a dietary restriction with increased physical activity was beneficial (Keys, 1980). Current research suggests just the opposite; the well-nourished patient tolerates treatment better and consequently tumour response to chemotherapy and radiation therapy improves. Furthermore, the interval between courses of treatment is reduced as there is no

Table 10.11

Weight (kg)	Age Approx.	Dosage							Provision							
		ml/kg/day					ml/day		per kg/day							
		VAMIN	20% I/L	15% Dex	Ped-El	Total Fluid	Vitlipid	Solivito	kCal	Fat (g)	Amino Acids (g)	CHO (g)	Na⁺ mmol	K⁺ mmol	Ca²⁺ mmol	Mg²⁺ mmol
20–30	6–12	30	15	25	5	75	4	10	57	3	1.8	6.7	1.5	1.3	0.82	0.125

Note:
Introduce regimen on a graded basis, over three days.
Calorie shortfall may be made up by (cautiously) increasing glucose infusion to 20% concentration, from 15% and/or raising dosage of fat to greater than 4 g/kg day.
To avoid ketosis, daily CHO intake (g/kg) must be more than, or at least equal to daily fat intake (g/kg).

need for protracted convalescence (Copeland and Dudrick, 1975). It has even been suggested that elective TPN reduces disease relapse when given in advanced neuroblastoma.

In conclusion, the most important aspect of nutritional care is early awareness and appropriate intervention. What may appear to be unpleasant and over-invasive procedures such as nasogastric feeding are often in both the short- and long-term interest of the child.

10.12 PAIN RELIEF

There are many misconceptions and myths about children's pain, their ability to express or describe it and about its management. Common myths include:

1. Children do not experience pain with the same intensity as adults because their nervous systems are different. In fact children's pain fibres may be more sensitive to pain than in adults (Haslam, 1969; Kaiko, 1980).
2. Children who are active cannot be in pain. Adults in pain may take to their beds but children may be up and about to distract themselves from pain or to avoid being 'caught' for pain relief, i.e. if pain relief is in the form of an intramuscular injection, the pain may seem preferable to the treatment.
3. Fear of children becoming addicted to narcotics. Often there is lack of knowledge by health care professionals about addiction, a myth dispelled by scientific data (Porter and Jick, 1980).
4. Fear of respiratory depression in children. Again due to lack of knowledge or experience. Narcotics are safe when administered in appropriate dosages and respiratory depression is almost unheard of when dose is titrated against pain levels.
5. Children will always tell you when they are in pain. If children equate pain relief with further pain, e.g. an injection, they may prefer not to admit to having pain. If the pain has been of gradual onset over a period of time they may have become 'used' to it and be unaware that it can be helped until it has been alleviated.
6. Children cannot tell you where the pain is. Children's age, development and vocabulary may limit their ability compared to adults. However, children as young as 18 months can localize and report their pain (McGrath, 1989).
7. The most effective way to control pain is by injection. This is probably the least satisfactory method and should be used only if and when other methods have been fully explored.
8. Parents are the best advisors on their child's pain and its control.

Although parents have a wealth of knowledge about their child, its ability to express pain and the usual effective method of controlling minor pains, the parents themselves may be stressed and anxious and therefore unable to help.

Types of pain

The pain experienced by children may be directly attributable to their disease and aggravated by the fears of coming into hospital. Five different types of cancer-related pain have been described (Mathews, Zarrow and Osterholm, 1973). Pain may be due to:

1. Nerve compression or invasion. Terms such as sharp, continuous, burning, boring, shock-like or searing may be used to describe it.
2. Bone destruction with infarction. Words like sharp, dull or a feeling of pressure may be used.
3. Infiltration of skin or tissue. This may lead to stretching sensations and dull aches that get progressively worse as the tumour grows.
4. Obstruction of the bowel, ureter, bile duct. This may start as dull or poorly localized pain or as colic with intermittent severe, sharp cramping pain with intervals of pain-free periods. The obstruction of vessels and venous engorgement leading to oedema may be described as dull and aching, turning to ischaemic pain if the arterial supply is impaired.
5. Inflammation due to infection or necrosis. Expressions of mild tenderness to excruciating pain potentially over the involved area may be used. If fever is present there may be complaints of generalized aches.

However, the majority of pain experienced by children with cancer is treatment related (Miser et al., 1987).

Pain assessment

To assess accurately a child's pain, nurses must possess knowledge about pain pathways, the child's cognitive and developmental level and the nature of the child's disease. Pain can be assessed by observing: (i) physiological changes, e.g. heart rate, blood pressure, respiratory rate, and palmar sweat response; (ii) behavioral changes, e.g. body movements, facial expressions, cries or (iii) descriptively, in terms of quality, intensity, location, duration and temporal pattern of the pain (McGrath, 1989).

Seven alternative methods of assessing children's pain have been described (Alder, 1990): (i) questioning, (ii) visual analogue scale, (iii) faces scale, (iv) poker chips, (v) X marks the spot, (vi) verbal scales, (vii) pain diary. It has been suggested that the visual analogue scale and the Eland Colour Tool are the two best methods for assessing pain in children

(Eland, 1985; Devine, 1990). Both are quick and can be used by any member of the team including the parents. It should be emphasized that pain assessment may not be fruitful if the method of pain relief is an intramuscular injection.

Pain relief

Once the type and degree of pain has been identified the method of pain relief must be addressed. There are a number of approaches available including pharmacological, psychological, anaesthetic blocks, TENS machines and the use of palliative chemotherapy and radiotherapy in the terminal care stage (Goldman, 1992). Management of the pain must be acceptable to the child and family. If the pharmacological approach is indicated the choice as to the method of pain relief includes the type of analgesic, dose and route. The use of flow sheets to record pain rating, vital signs, timing, dosage and administration of analgesia and other methods of pain relief assists evaluation of efficacy (Meinhart and McCaffery, 1983). It is important to remember that once pain relief is achieved the administration of further analgesia is *preventative*.

The choice of drug depends on the severity of pain; mild pain can be treated with non-narcotic analgesia, e.g. paracetamol and moderate pain with weak narcotics, e.g. dihydrocodeine, coproxamol. Severe pain requires narcotics, e.g. morphine, diamorphine. This approach has been described as the three-step progression or analgesic ladder (World Health Organisation, 1986). Non-steroidal anti-inflammatory agents, sedatives, antidepressants, anticonvulsants and steroids may have a role as an adjuvant form of therapy. Antidepressants and anticonvulsants have been found useful for neuropathic pain. Maximum tolerated doses must be

Table 10.12 Analgesia 'step ladder'

Step	<1	1–5	6–12	>12 years
1. Paracetamol p.o. 6 hourly	60–120 mg	120–250 mg	250–500 mg	500 mg–1 g
2. Dihydrocodeine p.o. 6 hourly	500 µg/kg	500 µg/kg	1 mg/kg	30 mg
or Codeine phosphate p.o. 4 hourly	←	0.5 mg/kg		→
3. Morphine p.o. 4 hourly	0.1 mg/kg	←	0.2 mg/kg	→
or Diamorphine i.v./s.c.	←	150 µg/kg stat 20–100 µg/kg/hr infusion		→

established before the efficacy of the drug is measured. When a calm reassuring environment and relationship is insufficient to calm a child psychotropic drugs may be required, e.g. diazepam, chlorpromazine or haloperidol. Analgesics should be prescribed regularly, according to their duration of action, not p.r.n. (see Table 10.12 for doses and schedules). When the oral route is not tolerated continuous infusions are preferable to intermittent bolus injections, as the level of analgesia is consistent. Subcutaneous infusions, using a local anaesthetic cream, are well tolerated and very effective. It is better to initially overestimate the intensity of the pain and subsequently reduce the analgesia as appropriate (Goldman, 1992). If the level of analgesia is insufficient or becomes inadequate the dose of morphine is titrated against the pain, increasing the dose by 30–50% until pain control is achieved.

MST is acceptable to many children as it is an oral preparation that only requires administration 12-hourly. While establishing effective levels of pain control short-acting morphine preparations are advisable for breakthrough pain.

Notes on opiate prescription

There is no such thing as a 'standard' dose of morphine.

To obtain control initially

The dose has to be adjusted for each child/adolescent until their pain is controlled. Prescribe an appropriate dose (usually give a range). Starting low and work up.

Use morphine tablets (Sevredol) or mixture for dose titration and give regularly every 4 hours.

At the same time prescribe the *same* dose for p.r.n. use for 'break-through' pain to be repeated as often as necessary.

Review after 24–48 hr and adjust regular dose according to break-through requirements. A common sequence of dose increments is (in mg):

5–10–15–20–30–40–60–80–100–120–150–200.

Once the patients are stable (and whenever possible for all patients before discharge home). Convert to twice-daily MST (controlled release morphine) tablets.

To calculate the MST dose, total the daily dose given as mixture or Sevredol tablets and divide by 2. Very few patients need to take MST more frequently than every 12 hours.

Routinely also prescribe morphine mixture or Sevredol tablets to have in case of breakthrough pain, at a dose equal to 1/6th of the total daily MST dose.

Parenteral opiate Use diamorphine instead of morphine because it is much more soluble.

Divide the dose of oral morphine by 3 to obtain the equianalgesic dose of diamorphine.

Clinical experience indicates that diamorphine is equipotent by *all* parenteral routes.

If frequent dosing is indicated consider continuous subcutaneous infusion.

Side effects

Side effects from opioids include constipation – laxatives should always be administered as opioids are commenced and sedation – this is common in children, particularly in the first 48 hours but gradually wears off. It is important to prepare parents for this to avoid fears that their child's condition is deteriorating. Dysphoria, respiratory and cough depression, nausea, urinary retention, biliary spasm and pruritus are also possible side effects but rarely limit the use of effective analgesics.

Shocked that their child requires such strong analgesics, parents may require help and support to accept pain relief in this form and reassurance that addiction is very rare.

REFERENCES

Alder S. (1990) Taking children at their word. Pain control in paediatrics. *Professional Nurse*. May, 398–402.

Antman, K.S., Griffin, J.D., Elias, A. *et al.* (1988) Effect of recombinant human granulocyte-macrophage colony-stimulating factor on chemotherapy-induced myelosuppression. *New England Journal of Medicine*, **319**, 593–598.

Brandt, S.J., Peters, W.P., Atwater, S.K. *et al.* (1988) Effect of recombinant human granulocyte-macrophage colony-stimulating factor on hematopoietic reconstitution after high-dose chemotherapy and autologous bone marrow transplantation. *New England Journal of Medicine*, **318**, 869–876.

Browne, M.J., Potter, D., Gress, J. *et al.* (1990) A randomized trial of open lung biopsy versus empiric antimicrobial therapy in cancer patients with diffuse pulmonary infiltrates. *Journal of Clinical Oncology*, **8**, 222–229.

Chopra, R., Fielding, A. and Goldstone, A.H. (1992) Successful treatment of fungal infections in neutropenic patients with liposomal amphotericin (AmBisome) – A report on 40 cases from a single centre. *Leukemia and Lymphoma*, **7**, 73–77.

Cohen, J. (1982) Antifungal chemotherapy. *Lancet*, **ii**, 532–537.

Cohen, J. and Glauser, M.P. (1991) Septic shock: treatment. *Lancet*, **338**, 736–739.

Copeland, E.M. and Dudrick, S. (1975) Cancer Nutritional Concepts. *Seminars in Oncology*, **2**, 329–335.

Devine, T. (1990) Pain management in paediatric oncology. *Paediatric Nursing*, Sept. 11–13.

DeWys, W.D. and Walters, K. (1975) Abnormalities of taste sensation in cancer patients. *Cancer*, **36**, 1888–1896.

DeWys, W.D. (1978) Changes in taste sensation and feeding behaviour in cancer patients: A review. *Journal of Homeopathic Nutrition*, **32**, 447–453.

Donaldson, S. (1977) Effect of nutrition as related to radiation and chemo-therapy, in *Nutrition and Cancer* (eds Myron Winick), John Wiley, New York, pp. 137–155.

Donaldson, S. (1982) Effects of therapy on nutritional status of the paediatric cancer patient. *Cancer Research*, **142**, 729.

Edwards, J.E. (1991) Invasive *Candida* infections. Evolution of a fungal pathogen. *New England Journal of Medicine*, **324**, 1060–1062.

Eland, J. (1985) The child who is hurting. *Seminars in Oncology Nursing*, **1**(2), 116–122.

Enno, A., Catovsky, D., Darrell, J. *et al.* (1978) Co-trimoxazole for prevention of infection in acute leukaemia. *Lancet*, **ii**, 395–397.

Glauser, M.P., Zanetti, G., Baumgartner, J.-D. *et al.* (1991) Septic shock: pathogenesis. *Lancet*, **338**, 732–736.

Golden, J.A., Chernoff, D., Hollander, H. *et al.* (1989) Prevention of *Pneumocystis carinii* pneumonia by inhaled pentamidine. *Lancet*, **i**, 654.

Goldman, A. (1992) Care of the dying child, in *Paediatric Oncology – Clinical Practice and Controversies* (eds P.N. Plowman and C.R. Pinkerton), Chapman & Hall, London.

Green, D.M., Finklestein, J.Z., Tefft, M.E. *et al.* (1989) Diffuse interstitial pneumonitis after pulmonary irradiation for metastatic Wilms' tumour. A report from the National Wilms' Tumour Study. *Cancer*, **63**, 450–453.

Guyton, A.C. (1976) *Textbook of Medical Physiology*, 5th edn. Saunders, Philadelphia.

Haas-Beckert, B. (1987) Removing the mysteries of parenteral nutrition. *Paediatric Nursing*, **13**(1), 37–41.

Haslam, D.R. (1969) Age and the perception of pain. *Psychonomic Science*, **15**, 86–87.

Hayes, F.A., Thompson, F.I., Hvizdala, E. *et al.* (1981) Chemotherapy as an alternative to laminectomy and radiation in the management of epidural tumor. *Journal of Pediatrics*, **104**, 221–224.

Hughes, W.T. (1987) *Pneumocystis carinii* pneumonitis. *New England Journal of Medicine*, **317**, 1021–1023.

Kaiko, R.F. (1980) Age and morphine analgesia in cancer patients with post operative pain. *Clinical Pharmacology Review*, **28**, 823–826.

Keys, A. (1980) *The Biology of Human Starvation*. Vols. I & II. North Central Publishing Co. St. Paul, Minn.

Leblanc, A., Caillaud, J.M., Hartmann, O. *et al.* (1984) Hypercalcemia pre-ferentially occurs in unusual forms of childhood non-Hodgkin's lymphoma, rhabdomyosarcoma, and Wilms' tumor. A study of 11 cases. *Cancer*, **54**, 2132–2136.

Lum, L.O. and Gallagher-Allred, C.R. (1984) Nutrition and the cancer patient: A co-operative effort by nursing and dietitians to overcome problems. *Cancer Nursing*, 469–474.

MacFadden, D.K., Edelson, J.D., Hyland, R.H. *et al*. (1987) Corticosteroids as adjunctive therapy in treatment of *Pneumocystis carinii* pneumonia in patients with acquired immunodeficiency syndrome. *Lancet*, **ii**, 1477–1479.

McGrath, P.A. (1989) Evaluating a child's pain. *Journal of Pain and Symptom Management*, **4**, 189–214.

Mathews, G., Zarrow, V. and Osterholm, J. (1973) Cancer pain and its treatment. *Seminars in Drug Treatment*, **3**, 45–53.

Meinhart, N.T. and McCaffery, M. (1983) *Pain – A Nursing Approach to Assessment and Analysis*, Norwalk, Conn. Appleton Century, p. 361.

Metcalf, D. (1989) Haemopoietic growth factors 1. *Lancet*, **i**, 825–827.

Miser J. *et al*. (1987) The presence of pain in a paediatric and young adult cancer population. *Pain*, **29**, 73–83.

Morton, A.R., Cantrill, J.A., Craig, A.E. *et al*. (1988) Single dose versus daily intravenous aminohydroxypropylidene biphosphonate (APD) for the hypercalcaemia of malignancy. *British Medical Journal*, **296**, 811–814.

Porter, J. and Jick, H. (1980) Addiction rate in patients treated with narcotics. *New England Journal of Medicine*, **303**, 123.

Shenep, J.L., Hughes, W.T., Robertson, P.K. *et al*. (1988) Vancomycin, ticarcillin and amikacin compared with ticarcillin-clavulanate and amikacin in the empirical treatment of febrile, neutropenic children with cancer. *New England Journal of Medicine*, **319**, 1053–1058.

Smit Veninga, K. (1985) Improving nutrition in children with cancer. *Paediatric Nursing*, **11**(1), 18–20.

Strohl, R.A. (1983) Nursing management of the patient with cancer experiencing taste changes. *Cancer Nursing*, **6**, 353–359.

Trogdon Wall, G. and Gabriel, L.A. (1983) Alterations of taste in children with leukaemia. *Cancer Nursing*, **6**, 447–452.

Westcott, W.B. *et al*. (1978) Alterations in whole saliva flow rate induced by fractionated radiotherapy. *American Journal of Roentgenology*, **130**, 145–149.

Wiley, J.M., Smith, N., Leventhal, B.G. *et al*. (1990) Invasive fungal disease in pediatric acute leukemia patients with fever and neutropenia during induction chemotherapy: A multivariate analysis of risk factors. *Journal of Clinical Oncology*, **8**, 280–286.

Woods, M. (1989) Tumour takes all. *Nursing Times*, **3**, 46–47.

World Health Organisation (1986) *Cancer Pain Relief*. WHO, Geneva, pp. 14–23.

Care of the dying child

Despite the success of the treatment of childhood cancer at least 30% will still die. Death from childhood cancer has changed, however, over the last 30–40 years. In the past children died quickly of their disease or complications of experimental treatment. Nursing care was supportive and not curative. Today most childhood cancer treatments offer the chance of hope and cure; however, this does mean from the time of diagnosis the child and his family are on an emotional 'roller coaster' as they go through periods of remission and relapse, enduring intense treatment protocols, perhaps still only to reach a terminal care stage.

Society finds the death of a child difficult to accept. It is angry and shocked, outraged that the death has disrupted the natural order of things (Judd, 1989). Despite the improvement in the cure rate of childhood cancer, many people still equate childhood cancer with death.

The challenges facing the multidisciplinary team to help the child and his family through this terminal stage are complex. They are faced not only with the physical and emotional care of the child but the psychological care of the whole family. The ability of the family and staff to cope through this stage reflects upon the extent of mutual trust that has developed between them over the course of the child's illness.

The majority of the deaths from cancer are from progression of the disease following months or years of gruelling treatment programmes. A small percentage, however, will be treatment related. These are often sudden and unexpected and therefore preparation for the death cannot always take place. Each family is unique, as is each family member. The ability to cope with the death of a child or sibling is dependent on many factors: (i) the development stage of the patient, (ii) the trusting relationship with the members of the health care team, (iii) the history of the child's treatment, (iv) the family's cultural and religious beliefs, and (v) the adaptive coping mechanisms of the family during the child's illness.

Health care professionals require an awareness of cultural diversities and the implications that they may have on the child and the family. Cultural attitudes and beliefs may influence how the family understands and reacts to the illness, treatment and death. The family's culture may affect the way they are able to trust the health care team, participate in the care and comply with treatment programmes and their restrictions. Problems or conflicts may occur for the medical team related to religious beliefs and treatment decisions, language or interpretation difficulties and beliefs of death and their rituals for death.

The decision to stop active treatment because cure or remissions are no longer achievable is not an easy one; it may be viewed as failure. The way in which this information is shared with families is important and may affect not only the way the family copes but is likely to remain a vivid lifetime memory (Woolley *et al.*, 1989). The information given to the family must not contain unrealistic hopes but at the same time must not leave them feeling abandoned.

Many factors influence the oncologist's decision to stop treatment. These may include: (i) the physical and emotional trauma experienced by the child during the treatment, (ii) the availability of second-line drugs, (iii) requests or urges from the parents or from the child to continue treatment, and (iv) the oncologist's own personal feelings. It must not be assumed that the parents understand and interpret the signs and symptoms of the child's disease in the same way that professionals do. Confirming that the disease has progressed is an unenviable task, however, as at the time of diagnosis the way in which information is shared with the parents will affect their ability to cope. Adequate preparation is vital. Details that parents have identified as having positive effects include: (i) both parents being spoken to together, (ii) privacy, (iii) uninterrupted time, (iv) the presence of a nurse, (v) the opportunity to ask questions, (vi) repetition and clarification of details, (vii) the opportunity to meet with the doctor again, and (viii) the opportunity to spend time alone together in private. Seeing parents together prevents one parent having to remember details accurately and then relay the bad news to their spouse, it avoids conflict if they interpret the information differently and prevents them feeling they have not been told everything. Single parents value the presence of a close friend or a nurse to provide the opportunity for discussion of the information and to clarify details.

Accepting the parents' and patient's grief is an important aspect for all members of the multidisciplinary team, to maintain trust and to build on future relationships.

If the child has not been present at the discussion confirming the relapse one issue that must be discussed quite quickly is how and when and who will tell the patient. The question of whether the child should know is no longer viable. Conflict arises between families when mutual pretence or concealed information is practised (Bluband Langer, 1978). The issue is how to tell the patient in a way that respects their complex coping ability. Parents feel reluctant to tell their child, worrying that their child will be unable to cope. Children's concepts of death are dependent upon their age, their level of development and their intellectual ability

(Spinetta, 1974). However, a child's ability to conceptualize death even at an early age can be accelerated when the child is faced with a life-threatening illness or death. If the child has been involved in the decision making about his treatment, and if he has had an honest and open relationship with his family and the multidisciplinary team, he will be at the same level of understanding.

The way in which information about the cessation of curative treatment and the plans for the future is discussed will vary depending upon the normal communication between family members. It should always be remembered that children are observant and can sense changes in parental emotions. If they feel their parents are unwilling or unable to discuss the results of the tests or other discussions with the doctors the conflicts of mutual pretence can begin. Children will adopt a role reversal and try to protect their parents and prevent causing additional emotional trauma by avoiding asking painful questions, even though they may have a great need to know. Trusting relationships with a particular member of the health care team may facilitate the patient to gain the information he wishes and have the opportunity to discuss it openly. Dilemmas can occur, however, if the parents are adamant that their child is not told the truth and ground rules may have to be established to enable parents and staff to work together through this conflict. Everyone including children has the right to know that they are dying but not everyone needs to know (Kubler Ross, 1970). Therefore we must strive to provide sufficient information in a conducive environment, so that when the child is ready he is able to ask questions or discuss issues that are important to him. Through therapeutic play, play therapists or psychologists are able to explore the feelings that children may be experiencing. Children's story books may facilitate opportunity to discuss fears, questions, anxieties or misconceptions the child may have about death and dying. Knowledge of these feelings or beliefs helps staff to meet the needs of the child more effectively. Providing children who are terminally ill with the opportunity to discuss issues related to death does not increase their death anxieties but decreases the feelings of isolation and alienation from the parents and other adults and may give the child reassurance that their illness is not too terrible to discuss. It is important to remember that individual beliefs, cultural and/or religious beliefs, are just that, individual. Families have their own beliefs and coping mechanisms and must feel comfortable in the way that they choose to deal with the situation. Discussing death and dying openly may be too painful for some families; if mutual pretence has been the family's normal way of handling things to change at this stage may be more alarming for the child. A member of the multidisciplinary team may adopt the role of communicator between the child and the family.

To enable the child to cope he needs to be involved in the planning of his care. Compliance depends upon an understanding of why and how, when and where. Even young children have unfulfilled wishes or requests to carry out and may want to have a say in their palliative treatment. Dilemmas may occur if the child refuses any further treatment and parents wish to pursue any chance of hope. Open discussion between the parents and the child may facilitate an answer to the conflict. Parents may feel they are giving up on their child if they do not explore every avenue; others, however, feel that their child may have already suffered enough physically or psychologically and to put them through more treatment is unacceptable. Hearing the reasons from the child for not undergoing more treatment may enable them to feel comfortable with the decisions. The child and the parents must not be left to feel that they are being abandoned. A child who is dying has to do so in a world of living children. Feelings of self-worth, self-respect and achievement are all important to the dying child. The need to reinforce the child's self-worth is necessary for planning terminal care. Goals should continue to be set and symptom control should facilitate the achievement of these. Achievement of goals enables the child to complete unfinished business and may be a way of ensuring being remembered, for example the distribution of personal toys and belongings amongst siblings and friends before their death. To prevent boredom and boost morale participation in normal daily routines, even attending school on a part-time basis should be encouraged (Lansky *et al.*, 1989).

11.1 SPIRITUAL ISSUES

Many nurses find it difficult to discuss spiritual issues with parents and children. Confusion occurs when spiritual and religious beliefs or needs are equated as the same. However, the fact that a person or family does not practise a religious faith does not mean that they do not have spiritual needs. Spiritual needs have been described as: (i) the need for meaning and purpose in life, (ii) the need to receive love, (iii) the need to give love, and (iv) the need for hope and creativity (Highfield and Carson, 1983). Although the chaplin is a member of the multidisciplinary team and is always available for the family and child, they will choose the person they wish to discuss their needs with. Nurses may feel uncomfortable but should utilize the resources available in the health care team to support the family and child as they face these issues.

11.2 SYMPTOM CONTROL

To provide effective symptom control nurses must possess knowledge about the physiology of childhood pain, the disease, its mode of spread and the psychological and physical implications that these may have for the child. Reviews and assessment must be carried out regularly so that treatments remain relevant and effective. Realistic goals of symptom control should be given to the child and family to avoid disappointment or distress and a loss of trust in the team if symptoms are not cured completely. A major fear of parents with a child with progressive disease is pain. The assessment and treatment of pain are discussed in Chapter 1. It should be remembered that health care professionals may believe that the parents are good judges or assessors of their child's pain; however, in the terminal stages there are factors that may influence their judgement, for example their own level of anxiety and stress may prevent them from recognizing their child's pain. The parents may also be relying on the nurses and doctors not to let their child suffer. Nursing documentation of previous effective methods of pain relief during treatment or at the time of diagnosis will be valuable. It is important that the method of pain relief is acceptable to the child and the parents. The parents may have difficulty agreeing to narcotic drugs at this stage, they may see this as accepting that their child is going to die, they may fear that strong drugs will hasten the end or that if started so soon they will not be strong enough at the end. Parents will require support and guidance to come to terms with these decisions.

Other methods of pain control that may be appropriate in the terminal stages include the use of chemotherapy. Symptoms from leukaemia cells in the central nervous system can be relieved by the use of intrathecal drugs and steroids.

Radiation has also been used to alleviate symptoms due to bony metastases, obstruction, spinal cord compression and local recurrences in skin and soft tissue. Anaesthetic blocks may be of value but are rarely used in paediatrics.

Cutaneous stimulation has a long history. For centuries mothers have been rubbing/massaging aches and pains as a first approach to pain control. Other approaches include heat or cold packs and recently TENS machines (transcutaneous electrical nerve stimulators). Local applications of cold or ice packs are thought to reduce muscle spasm and will also reduce inflammation (Lehmann and de Lateur, 1982).

It has been suggested that TENS machines produce pain relief by either (i) the electrical stimulation of larger peripheral nerve fibres 'closing the gate' preventing painful stimuli to the spinal cord cells or (ii) the electrical stimulation triggers the release of the patient's own endorphins (Caswell and Eland, 1989). The siting of the area to be stimulated can vary and patients and parents may have to adopt a flexible trial and error approach. Areas include directly over the pain, between two sites of pain, beyond, contralateral to the pain, acupuncture points or any site distal to the pain (McCaffery, 1990).

Relaxation and hypnotherapy has proved to be beneficial to children undergoing painful procedures during their treatment, both in relieving pain and reducing anxiety and therefore should be considered in the terminal phase (Zeltzer and Le Baron, 1982). Again this is a method of pain control that children can use themselves; it is particularly useful where children have intermittent episodes of breakthrough pain, where increasing the level of analgesia would result in unwanted side effects. It is also useful in relieving parents' anxieties if they participate in the process of relaxation.

Bleeding

This may be due to thrombocytopenia or coagulopathy caused by disease in the bone marrow or the myelosuppressive effects of treatment. Criteria for the administration of platelets during active treatment programmes may no longer be applicable in the terminal stages. At this time platelets are only administered if there are bleeding problems which interfere with the quality of the child's life. This should be discussed with the parents and the child so that they are aware that the criteria have changed. Administering red cell transfusions should be to improve or maintain a good quality of life. Tranexamic acid has been found to be of use in reducing spontaneous bleeds (Chambers *et al.*, 1989).

Nausea and vomiting

This may be due to raised intracranial pressure, chemotherapy, intestinal obstruction, compression of the stomach by a mass or analgesia. Previous knowledge and records of useful anti-emetics for chemotherapy will be valuable; haloperidol is useful as it is compatible with opioids and can be given in combination via a syringe pump. Cyclizine is of use when nausea is due to raised intracranial pressure and can also be given in combination with opioids. Metoclopramide should be avoided when the cause of the vomiting is intrinsic obstruction but may be useful when vomiting occurs due to external compression of intestine.

Dyspnoea

This may be due to disease in the lungs or a disease in the abdomen pressing on the diaphragm. Relief of this symptom includes a combination oxygen administration, opiates and the positioning of the patient. Suction and a humidified environment may also be of value in some cases.

Anorexia

This may be due to swallowing difficulties, mouth sores, nausea and vomiting or apathy about eating. Nutrition is covered in Chapter 10. Intervention at this stage should be aimed to maintain the patient's comfort. Parents need support to accept that total parenteral intervention or enteral feeding may not be appropriate.

Constipation

This may be due to inactivity, poor nutrition, chemotherapy or analgesics. Stool softeners such as lactulose and doxusate may be used in combination with stimulants such as bisacodyl and danthron. Children who have incomplete obstruction due to pressure of tumour require stool softeners to facilitate their bowels being opened; they may also require additional pain relief, for example Entonox, to control spasmodic pain as their bowels are activated.

Itching

This may be due to limited fluid intake, increased cachexia, analgesics or jaundice. Patients may obtain relief of symptoms using antihistamines and topical steroids or menthol creams may be of value. If the cause is an opioid it may be necessary to change to a different drug.

Insomnia and restlessness

This may be due to bladder or bowel distension which may be helped by long acting morphine at night, with or without chlorpromazine.

Muscle twitching in the terminal stages

The cause is unknown but diazepam, chlorpromazine or haloperidol have been found to be of use.

Noisy respiration (death rattle)

This is due to the accumulation of secretions in the posterior pharynx. Regular hyoscine has been found to be useful on occasions, as has gentle suction using soft suction catheters if it is acceptable to the patient.

Seizures

These may be due to primary or metastatic disease of the central nervous system. Anticonvulsants as appropriate will be used; however the parents will need support and advice to cope with a seizure, especially if they are at home. Supplies of diazepam with instructions for its use are advisable if the parents wish to care for their child at home if convulsions are a possibility.

11.3 HOME CARE/HOSPITAL

Choosing where their child should die is a decision that is difficult for parents to make. Home care for the dying child is recognized to be both feasible and desirable. It has been demonstrated that there are benefits to the child, the parents and the rest of the family when the death takes place in the home (Martinson, 1978).

Parents require support and information to make the decision to take their child home to die. There are factors that may influence them, including the distance from the hospital, the resources available from the hospital and those available in the community, the duration of the terminal illness and the quality of the child's life. Parents need help and support to make each day that the child has left count. The same high quality of management and care should be practised regardless of where the terminal phase takes place.

As a general practitioner (GP) is likely only to ever see one or two cases of childhood cancer it is unlikely that they will be experienced in supporting a child and family during their terminal stage. Effective communication and links are, therefore, vital to enable the GP and their team to support this family. The majority of paediatric oncology units in the UK have their own community liaison nurse or team to coordinate the help available in the community, acting as a resource and educator to the community health care team. Joint visits by the hospital carers and community staff help reassure the parents that close communication is taking place. Paediatric hospices who offer respite care may be appropriate for some children with cancer where the death is protracted and the whole family require respite care.

If the child's condition necessitates that the death occurs in hospital, or if the parents choose to stay in hospital, they will require support to adjust to the process of dying in a public place. Some parents may find staying on the ward very supportive, being surrounded by other parents with whom they have developed unique support and coping mechanisms. However, in the terminal stages these networks may be severely tested. Every parent will be reminded that death is a possibility and may question the outcome if their child is receiving similar treatment as the one who is dying.

It is a testing time for members of the multidisciplinary team, trying to create an environment that encourages hope and support for those patients who are newly diagnosed and support for those preparing for death. How and what to tell other patients on the ward may be difficult for some of the parents and members of the staff. Children are astute observers and pick up cues from adult conversation, behaviour and body language. Creating feelings of mutual pretence that nothing unusual is happening create feelings of mistrust which may leave the patients frightened. Children require appropriate information and an opportunity with someone they trust to discuss or ask questions about the dying child. This is particularly important if that child has the same diagnosis as they may wish to express feelings and fears about the implications for their own treatment and perhaps death. Structured play sessions may facilitate these discussions about death.

Questions that are frequently and repeatedly asked by the parents include 'how will he die? will I know when he is dead? what do I do when he is dead?' Answers based upon the child's current status require sensitivity and honesty that appropriately reassure the parents. It is impossible to completely prepare parents for the death of their child. Even up to the time of death parents continue to hope that it will not happen. They may be frightened to leave their child in case they die while they are away.

Parents may never have discussed funeral arrangements for their child with each other before and may have different views. To discuss this after the child's death when they are emotionally raw may result in decisions being made that they later regret. Occasionally the child himself may wish to be involved in this discussion. Equally, decisions about clothes to be worn after the death ensures that a special outfit can be available. Parents may also want to discuss their role in the final preparation after death. When the child has died the parents may experience many mixed emotions. As much as they wanted their child to live they wanted him to do so as a normal healthy child and therefore may have felt prolonging the death was only extending the pain and suffering. They may feel relieved, relieved that their child is no longer suffering, that their ordeal is over. However, they may feel guilty for feeling relieved. They may be very shocked by the death, even though they thought they were prepared for it. When the child has died parents may prefer to spend time alone with their child. This may enable them to achieve a feeling of finality. It provides the opportunity to say parting words and see their child lying peacefully, suffering no more indignities or pain.

After the death the final preparation should be carried out in accordance with the parents' wishes. Some parents may feel the need to rush away from the hospital, while others are very reluctant to go and should be made to feel welcome for as long as they feel the need to stay. Leaving the hospital without their child is a very painful and difficult experience. Arrangements for the family to be taken home, unless the parents do not wish it, should be made. Parents may request a special nurse to stay with their child and escort him from the ward, or they may wish to carry or escort their own child to the hospital chapel to help in the process of leaving the ward.

It is important that the GP and community team are informed of the child's death as soon as possible.

11.4 SIBLINGS

Siblings of children with cancer require direct information about the disease and the implications of the treatment and the outcome (Lindsay and McCarthy, 1974; Kagen-Goodheart, 1977). Education and effective communication have been demonstrated to improve in the way siblings cope. The grief experienced by the parents of a dying child cannot be hidden from the siblings. As previously mentioned, children are astute observers and will pick up cues from adult conversation, behaviour and body language. They may be frightened and confused but again avoid asking questions that may upset their parents. Siblings may well experience fear that it is something they have wished upon their sibling or something that might also happen to them. Feelings of jealousy for all the attention their sick sibling receives are also experienced.

Involving the siblings minimizes the feelings of isolation from the family and establishes an atmosphere of honesty and openness. As with the ill patient if the sibling has been involved throughout the treatment programme they will be aware of the implications of relapse and no further active treatment. Explanations of the decisions and goals made by the family and medical team should be given at an appropriate level for the developmental stage of the sibling. Parents may express feelings that the siblings cannot cope and should not know. However, studies have shown that siblings who were not informed or involved experienced emotional problems including unresolved feelings of guilt, remorse or fear of death two to three years after the death of their sibling (Spinetta *et al.*, 1981). The siblings will be the long-term survivors, they have unique needs of their own and need help to cope with and adjust to the death of their sibling. They may have important things to say and do with their brother or sister before they die.

Issues the parents may need help to deal with are – should siblings be present at the death? should they see their dead sibling? and should they attend the funeral? It should be up to the individual sibling; they may wish to have the opportunity to spend time alone with their dead sibling to speak to them in private, they may wish to say goodbye at the funeral. It is important that it is their choice; it is not something they feel they should or should not do. They will need support, reassurance and explanations to make their decision. To support the child in case the parents are unable to, it has been found helpful to have a significant person for the siblings who will care for them and leave with them when they are ready.

Returning to school during the terminal phase or after the death may be difficult and painful for the well sibling. Visits by members of the health care team are useful to prepare the teachers and classmates to cope and be supportive and understanding.

11.5 GRANDPARENTS

Supporting grandparents is a difficult but important task. By virtue of their age and experience in life society assumes grandparents can cope and should be experienced with death. This is not always true. They also have the additional burden of grieving not only for their grandchild but for their child as well. Involving them in the care, or providing them with a role and a purpose helps them to cope and may reduce some of the anxiety that the parents themselves have about their own parents.

11.6 STAFF SUPPORT

Nursing staff establish unique relationships with the children and their families. This is particularly true during the terminal stage when everyone is striving to meet all the emotional and physical needs. Team work is vital to provide a supportive environment where feelings of anger, frustration, denial, guilt and sadness can be shared.

11.7 BEREAVEMENT AND MOURNING

When a child dies the parents may enter a period of grief which is extended, intense and slow to resolve. The phases of grief that parents may experience include: (i) a period of numbness and shock, (ii) a period of intense grief, and (iii) a period of reorganization or recovery (Parkes, 1986). During the period of numbness and shock parents may find it difficult to make decisions about everyday occurrences, others carry on as if nothing has happened. As the numbness lifts parents may experience feelings of anger, guilt, panic, pain and depression. They search for a meaning or a reason as to why the death happened and yearn for the dead child. During this time they often neglect their own basic physical needs, which may result in their own health suffering. It is important to remember that reorganization is not recovery. Many parents doubt that they will reach a stage of reorganization. However, a time does come when parents realize the good days outnumber the bad days and they will have enthusiasm and energy for other things in their life. Memories about the child become happy and enriched. There are days, however, which create anxieties for the parents, such as anniversaries, birthdays of the dead child, Christmas and other family occasions. Parents require support and advice to be able to make the day enjoyable for their other children and allow them time to grieve for their dead sibling. Mourning has been described as 'not forgetfulness but enriched remembrance' (Cantor, 1978). The need to talk and reminisce about their child continues long after the death. Sadly society expects parents to get over it quickly. They feel uncomfortable and avoid conversations with the parents for risk of upsetting them. Bereavement facilities available from the hospital or within the community should be identified to the parents at the appropriate time. Bereavement groups, counsellors and parents' self-help groups may be of use and benefit to some parents.

Terminally ill children deserve the optimal care by compassionate and competent carers. Careful planning can prevent or effectively control symptoms, leaving the parents with a bearable memory of a quiet peaceful death.

In all cultures children are particularly valued and seen as society's hopes, dreams and future (Bandman and Bandman, 1985).

REFERENCES

Bandman, E. and Bandman, B. (1985) *Nursing Ethics in the Life Span*. Appleton-Century-Crofts, Norwalk, Conn.

Bluebond-Langer, M. (1978) *The Private World of Dying Children*. Princeton University Press.

Cantor, R.C. (1978) *And a Time to Live. Toward Emotional Well Being during the Crisis of Cancer*. Harper & Row, New York.

Caswell, L. and Eland, J. (1989) Don't bump my bed, don't touch my feet. *Journal of American Pediatric Oncology Nursing*, **6**(4), 111–120.

Chambers, E.J., Oakhill, A., Cornish, J.M. *et al.* (1989) Terminal care at home for children with cancer. *British Medical Journal*, **298**, 937–940.

Highfield, M.F. and Carson, C. (1983) Spiritual needs of patients: are they recognised? *Cancer Nursing*, **6**, 3.

Judd, D. (1989) *Give Sorrow Words*. Free Association Books, London.

Kagen-Goodheart L. (1977) Living with childhood cancer. *American Journal of Orthopsychiatry*, **47**(4), 651–658.

Kubler-Ross, E. (1970) *On Death and Dying*. Tavistock Press, London.

Lansky, S.B., Ritter-Sterr, C. and List, M.A. (1989) Psychiatric and psychological support of the child and adolescent with cancer, in *Principles and Practice of Paediatric Oncology* (eds P.A. Pizzo and D.G. Poplack) Lippincott, Philadelphia.

Lehmann, J.F. and de Lateur, B.J. (1982) *Cryotherapy: Therapeutic Heat and Cold* (ed J.F. Lehmann) 3rd edn, Williams & Wilkins, Baltimore, pp. 563–602.

Lindsay, M. and McCarthy, S. (1974) Caring for the brothers and sisters of a dying child, in: *Care of the Child facing Death* (ed L. Burton) Routledge & Kegan Paul, Boston.

Martinson, I. (1978) Home care for children dying of cancer. *Paediatrics*, **62**, 106–113.

McCaffery, M. (1990) Nursing approaches to nonpharmacological pain control. *International Journal of Nursing Studies*, **27**(1), 1–5.

Parkes, C.M. (1986) *Bereavement: Studies of Grief in Adult Life*, New York International Universities Press, Inc.

Spinetta, J.J. (1974) The dying child's awareness of death. *Psychology Bulletin*, **81**(4), 256–260.

Spinetta, J.J., Swarne, J.A. and Sheposh, J.P. (1981) Effective parental coping following the death of a child from cancer. *Journal of Paediatric Psychology*, **6**, 251–263.

Woolley, H., Stein, A., Forrest, G.C. *et al.* (1989) Imparting the diagnosis of life threatening illness in children. *British Medical Journal*, **298**, 1623–1626.

Zeltzer, L. and Le Baron, S. (1982) Hypnosis and nonhypnotic techniques for reduction of pain and anxiety during painful procedures in children and adolescents with cancer. *Behavioural Paediatrics*, **101**(6), 1032–1035.

12 | The long-term survivor of childhood cancer

In the past cancer was synonymous with death and thus the psychosocial care of the child with cancer and his family was directed at preparing the family for the death of their child. With advances in treatment, the focus has moved to include long-term effects in the child receiving treatment for their cancer (Pinkerton, 1992).

It is now estimated that in the year 2000 approximately 1 in every 1000 young adults will be a survivor of childhood cancer (Meadows and Hobbie, 1986). Thus the psychosocial and late medical effects in the long-term survivor of childhood cancer and his family are now important considerations to be included in total patient care.

12.1 SPECIFIC MEDICAL SEQUELAE

Treatment-related sequelae may be due to any of the three main therapeutic modalities: chemotherapy, radiation or surgery. As discussed earlier, with improved preoperative chemotherapy, mutilating surgical procedures can now be avoided in the majority of patients and major surgical sequelae should be a thing of the past. Long-term complications from chemotherapy and irradiation are often due to an interaction of the two, particularly where high-dose radiotherapy is combined with alkylating agents. Radiation-related growth defects may be direct or indirect. Following treatment of orbital rhabdomyosarcoma in the younger child there will be considerable facial asymmetry due to direct radiation-induced under-development of the orbital bone, muscle and soft tissue (Figure 12.1). Hemi-abdominal irradiation for Wilms' tumour will produce under-development of soft tissue and musculature. A similar effect is seen in the neck following irradiation for cervical Hodgkin's disease and it is for this reason that bilateral irradiation is used for unilateral, high cervical disease. Spinal shortening due to irradiation on vertebral bodies is an important problem in children treated for medulloblastoma or CNS leukaemia. In the past inclusion of only part of the vertebral body in

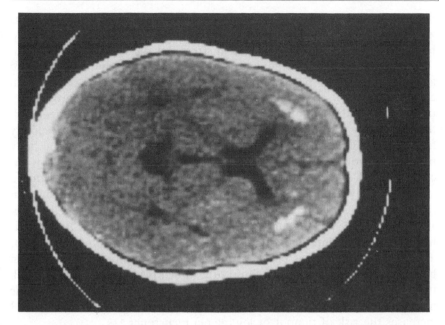

Figure 12.1 CT scan of brain following radiotherapy and intrathecal methotrexate. Typical intracerebral calcification associated with leucoencephalopathy is seen.

unilateral abdominal irradiation for Wilms' tumour led to considerable scoliosis due to asymmetrical body growth. Irradiation fields which include the hip, e.g. for Ewing's sarcoma, may result in aseptic necrosis or slipped femoral epiphyses. Inclusion of the long bone epiphyses in younger children will lead to growth arrest and limb asymmetry and irradiation to the diaphyseal region may result in abnormal bone modelling. Abnormal dentition is a consequence of treatment to the jaw with blunted roots, decreased calcification and delayed or arrested development. There may also be trismus and jaw malocclusion. These effects are all related to the total dose of radiation given and the age at which the child is treated (Probert, Parker and Kaplan, 1973; Brown *et al.*, 1983; Wallace *et al.*, 1990).

Linear growth will also be indirectly affected by the influence of radiation on hormonal function. Abnormal growth of children with cancer is often multifactorial involving subtle abnormalities in hypothalamic/pituitary function, thyroid function, the effect of steroid treatment, malnutrition, chronic illness and psychological factors. There is, however, clear evidence that cranial irradiation at doses as low as 18 Gy produces abnormalities of growth hormone (GH) production due either to an effect on the pituitary gland or on hypothalamic production of growth hormone releasing factor (Kirk *et al.*, 1987; Clayton *et al.*, 1988). Many patients who show no evidence of growth velocity retardation have been shown to have blunted GH responses to insulin stress test or arginine provocation. Abnormal patterns of unstimulated pulsatile growth hormone release are also described. The precise indications for treatment with GH remain controversial, but if one waits until there is demonstrable growth retardation GH administration may only have a marginal benefit. In general, therefore, any child who has had cranial irradiation must be closely followed up. Those with brain tumours or who have received total body irradiation should attend special growth clinics, jointly reviewed by oncologists and paediatric endocrinologists. Any suggestion of reduced growth velocity necessitates evaluation of hypothalamo-pituitary function (Sanders *et al.*, 1986). If this is abnormal GH therapy should be considered (Milner, 1986; Lannering and Albertsson-Wiklund, 1987). It is likely that such intervention will prevent further decline in growth, although if the spine has been irradiated growth hormone administration has no effect on sitting height. Slow virus infections have been linked with the use of human GH but this is no longer a problem with the synthetic hormone currently used. There is also no convincing evidence that GH increases the risk of tumour or leukaemia recurrence.

Complex hypothalamic dysfunction syndromes may lead to early puberty or delayed puberty. Early onset of puberty may minimize the value of GH administration due to premature fusion of the epiphyses and there may be an indication for delaying puberty with adminstration of gonadotrophin releasing hormone analogues (Leiper *et al.*, 1987). Thyroid dysfunction is often demonstrable in children who have received irradiation for cervical Hodgkin's lymphoma (Schimpff *et al.*, 1980). Many will have elevated TSH levels but be asymptomatic and have normal T3/T4 levels. Thyroxine supplementation is generally recommended for such patients in order to avoid TSH-induced nodular hyperplasia and possible late malignancy (Moroff and Fuks, 1986).

Neurological sequelae resulting from whole brain irradiation has been extensively studied. There are major difficulties in evaluating this because a variety of psychological factors will contribute to any abnormalities detected (Larcombe *et al.*, 1990). It does seem clear, however, that there is a small but significant decline in IQ and subtle deficits in areas of learning, such as numeracy (Jannoun, 1983; Copeland *et al.*, 1988; Appleton *et al.*, 1990). This has been used as an argument for replacing irradiation with more intensive intrathecal chemotherapy or the addition of high dose systemic methotrexate in ALL, although the late toxicity of the latter remains to be clarified. Minor learning abnormalities should be compensatable by awareness amongst teachers and early intervention. Patients who have received more than one course of cranial irradiation, e.g. due to CNS relapse, total body irradiation preceding bone marrow transplant procedures or high doses for brain tumours, run a risk of more significant complications. Leucoencephalopathy with intracranial calcification, and cerebral atrophy on CT scan and MRI, occur and seizure disorders may result (Ochs *et al.*, 1983; Packer *et al.*, 1986) (Figure 12.2).

Treatment-related infertility is an issue frequently raised by parents. Irradiation of ovaries and testes, even at small doses, will produce infertility but there are rarely indications for this, one exception being testicular relapse in ALL. Alkylating agents, such as cyclophosphamide, chlorambucil, and procarbazine will almost invariably cause sterility in boys but the ovary is considerably more resistant and long-term follow-up studies have shown that most girls retain fertility (Kreuser *et al.*, 1988; Aubier *et al.*, 1989). The Leydig cells of the testis are chemoresistant, unlike the germinal epithelium, and problems with secondary sex characteristics are uncommon.

Other organs

Late tissue effects may be the sequelae of earlier acute toxicity or be primary complications that have delayed onset (Perry and Yarbro, 1984).

The cardiac toxicity of anthracyclines has been known for many years but until recently it was thought to be relatively safe to give a cumulative dose of up to $350–400\,mg/m^2$. Patients who had had prior mediastinal irradiation or whole lung irradiation were known to be at increased risk.

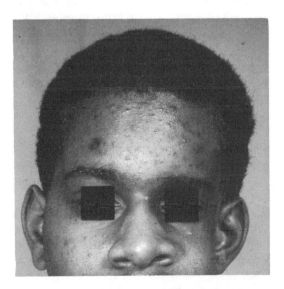

Figure 12.2 Facial asymmetry associated with irradiation of a Ewing's sarcoma of the zygomatic bone at the age of 3 years.

Recent studies, however, have suggested that the safe limit is much lower, if indeed it exists at all (Lipshultz *et al.*, 1991; Yeung *et al.*, 1991). Even with doses of less than $100 \, mg/m^2$ detailed echocardiographic studies have shown some evidence of cardiac dysfunction. This adverse effect appears to be related to young age and subsequent cardiac growth. Less commonly, cardiac effusions, pericarditis and premature coronary artery disease may occur in patients who have received high total doses. The problem is that this toxicity may present very late, even 10–20 years after initial chemotherapy. Patients have been known to die due to sudden cardiac failure during heavy exercise with no forewarning symptoms. Alternatively, the patient presents with clinical signs of cardiac failure such as dyspnoea and hepatomegaly. The damage is irreversible and although in mild to moderate cases cardiac function may be supported with drugs such as digoxin the outcome is usually poor. Cardioxane chelates the free iron which forms a toxic complex with anthracycline in cardiac muscle and its administration with the anthracycline may reduce toxicity (Speyer *et al.*, 1988). New anthracycline analogues such as epirubicin and idarubicin may have less cardiac toxicity, although this has not been clearly demonstrated in children.

Bleomycin is an important cause of pulmonary toxicity, producing interstitial fibrosis and demonstrable reduction in CO transfer factor. This effect is dose related and more common with weekly administration schedules. High oxygen concentrations under general anaesthesia may predispose to damage. The drug is now less commonly used and should be avoided if possible. BCNU has been implicated as a cause of chronic pulmonary dysfunction in children with brain tumours. When used at very high dose with autologous bone marrow rescue this drug causes an acute pneumonitis.

Chronic liver disease may result from methotrexate-induced hepatotoxicity or chronic graft versus host disease after allogeneic bone marrow transplant.

Cataracts are almost inevitable after irradiation of the orbit for rhabdomyosarcoma or retinoblastoma and there is also a high incidence after total body irradiation.

Second tumours

It is a cruel fact that up to 10% of cancer patients will develop a second malignancy as a result of their treatment. Moreover, recent intensification of treatment regimens may further increase the likelihood of this. Predisposing syndromes, such as retinoblastoma, neurofibromatosis, naeval basal cell carcinoma and xeroderma pigmentosa may contribute in a small number. In general, the complication is dose related, as in the case of second bone tumours following irradiation for soft-tissue sarcoma, or retinoblastoma. There is a clear link with the administration of alkylating agents, the highest incidence being in Hodgkin's disease where a combination of alkylating agents plus irradiation is involved. Acute myeloid leukaemia is the commonest haematological second tumour, although ALL and Hodgkin's disease have also been reported. Second solid tumours, apart from bone tumours, include a variety of soft-tissue sarcomas (Ingram et al., 1987; Kushner, Zauber and Tan, 1988; Tucker et al., 1988; de Vathaire et al., 1989).

Recently the epipodophyllotoxins teniposide and etoposide have been implicated in the development of secondary myeloid leukaemia. This effect is both dose and schedule related and appears to be linked with a specific chromosome translocation in leukaemia cells involving chromosome 21q23 (Pui et al., 1991).

12.2 PSYCHOSOCIAL ASPECTS

Questions which are raised include: What are parents' concerns as treatment is completed and remission lengthens? How will the family cope with any chronic illness? Who determines which family requires additional support and perhaps counselling and at what stage should intervention take place?

Psychosocial problems in adjusting to the child with cancer may already have been detected in some families, to the degree that intervention with counselling may already be established. These sessions will obviously continue until completion of their specialist treatment and close follow-up.

The completion of treatment may, however, bring with it many concerns, questions and anxieties which need consideration and, if not addressed, may allow preventable or early detectable long-term sequelae to pass unnoticed.

Research into psychosocial long-term effects of surviving childhood cancer (which includes parents) is limited. The most detailed study is by Drs Koocher and O'Malley in their work entitled *The Damocles Syndrome*. Although their study was first published in 1981, much can still be gained from consideration of their findings.

Parents

The impact of the diagnosis of cancer for the parents of a child is often expressed as indescribable. Parents do not expect their child to be facing a life-threatening illness before themselves or their parents. For many parents, although the risk of relapse during their child's treatment does exist, they mainly feel 'safe' for the duration of the treatment. Thus, when treatment has been completed, the expected feelings of a sense of achievement and relief are often tainted by the 'bittersweet' (Wofford, 1987) negative feelings of 'what now?' and the fear of recurrence.

On completion of their child's treatment the parents (sometimes more so than previously) required help and support and yet this is the time when support is being withdrawn (Koocher and O'Malley, 1981; Wallace, Reiter and Pendergrass, 1987). The reassurance and security of hospital visits become less frequent as remission time increases. The assumption that the longer the remission the lower the anxiety levels for these parents is not borne out. In fact the reverse appears to be the case. Many parents reported feelings of abandonment once their child's treatment had been completed.

Koocher and O'Malley's research study describes the responses of 103 parents of children who are long-term survivors. Wallace, Reiter and Pendergrass also conducted a study and both reported strikingly similar findings. These include parental fears about:

1. Long-term sequelae of treatment, especially the possibility of development of a second malignancy.
2. Their child's physical condition.
3. The child's ability to maintain relationships with the opposite sex in later life and marriage worries.
4. The child's ability to have children.
5. Employment discrimination.
6. The child's emotional development and their relationship with siblings, peers and other members of the family.

Aside from these anxieties, many parents reported that follow-up appointments were very stressful, with the build-up a week or so prior to the appointment equally stressful. Fear of what they might be told and the uncertainty of recurrence were at the forefront.

In both these studies, parents made suggestions to the health care workers of suggested interventions which may benefit future parents. They would have liked additional information and support. Approximately 60% reported that they had considered seeking information but the channels by which to do this were not made obvious. Parents reported needing regular progress reports on their children which were of a factual nature.

Written material regarding potential problems their children may experience after ceasing treatment should be made readily available. Some parents felt that an education programme for themselves and their child may be useful, although others found this concept undesirable.

Although follow-up appointments might only be yearly, parents wanted to be able to have regular contact with their oncology centre if needed and to feel comfortable in asking for additional appointments if wanted. They also felt that additional help to support themselves should be available, which should include financial support and emotional assessment of their ability to cope with resources available to deal with any problems.

One suggestion for the support and educational programme was to ask parents of children who are longer-term survivors than themselves to meet with them. The diagnosis and age of the child survivor should be similar to their child's. Two-thirds of these parents said they would consider being a contact parent for future parents and they suggested the introduction should be early in the diagnosis and treatment.

Although appreciating the difficulty in not treating their child as 'special' at diagnosis and during intensive treatments, the parents advise that other parents should try to treat their child as though they are going to survive. They strongly advise against over-indulgence and over-protection, both of which can produce long-term problems.

Lastly, parents were asked what they considered important in helping them cope with their experience. The reply was the need for accurate, frequent and honest communication. Many parents felt that they would have benefited from a psychological referral within a week of the diagnosis of their child. They felt that, although family and members of the medical/nursing team were very supportive, their primary concern was, appropriately, for the child. Although the care givers recognize the need for parents to express their feelings, the parents were acutely aware that this was time consuming in their already busy schedule. They also felt that a referral at the beginning of treatment for all parents ruled out the stigma of a later referral.

Koocher (1985) in his work 'Psychological Care of the Child Cured of Cancer' states the importance of assessing families for the stresses and anxieties related to the psychological aspects of survivorship. He recommends that families should be assessed at regular intervals which would lead to detecting those families who may develop psychological maladjustment.

Children

Regardless of age, any child diagnosed with cancer will exhibit some manifestations of depression, separation anxieties, worries and fears of the unknown.

Studies of long-term survivors of childhood cancer reviewing the psychosocial aspects have different conclusions regarding the lengths of these reactions. Lansky et al. (1985) states that the patients have an interruption in their development and do not overcome this problem. Koocher and O'Malley's (1981) study of long-term childhood survivors report an adjustment problem in 47%.

Regardless of the percentages of psychosocial maladjustment, they do exist and must be recognized. In Koocher and O'Malley's study 117 long-term childhood cancer survivors were interviewed. Long term in this study was defined as five years since the diagnosis. They examined individual issues such as marriage, children, employment and adjustment in the light of physical/visible impairment. They also identified ways in which survivors reacted to the stresses of long-term survivorship.

Reaction to the stress of the diagnosis of cancer was found to be age related. In more than one study it was demonstrated that the younger the age of diagnosis the less likely there is to be long-term psychosocial sequelae. It is thought that at these very young ages of infancy and early childhood the patient is unable to verbalize their experience and many have no memory of it. However, the age at which they were informed of their previous cancer history also affected long-term adjustment problems. The younger they were told about their previous diagnosis and experience, the fewer adjustment problems they developed.

For those aware of their history and who had memories of the experience the reaction to this stress was in one of three ways:

1. Preoccupation with the disease, with the conviction that the disease will return and prove fatal.
2. Belief that the treatment already received had protected them, for life, against further insult of the cancer.
3. Coping well with the uncertainty of the disease by 'not worrying about it'.

The first group showed significant levels of anxiety and had other psychological problems. The second group and a few of the third group denied the potential late effects of treatment. They would, conversely, be overburdened with any late effects of treatment having failed to face up to these gradually. Failure to attend out-patient follow-up appointments is not uncommon with these patients. Prevention or early intervention of side effects is missed and this group manifest greater anxieties and depressions, shown by the following behaviour: Fear of failure; increased dependence of parents; social immaturity; poor self-image; lack of confidence and difficulty in maintaining peer relationships or relationships with the opposite sex. These survivors experience lack of self-esteem, loss of orientation to life and an inability to plan their future.

Self-esteem, defined as 'extent to which a person believes himself or herself worthy, capable and significant' (Gilberts, 1983) develops from a very early age and is affected by life's experiences. An interruption to this development by a life-threatening illness can result in regression and dependence. Greenberg, Kazak and Meadows (1989) and Koocher and O'Malley report that children who have survived cancer have lower self-esteem than similar groups of well children. The importance of self-esteem is described by Reasoner (1983) and its importance in achieving a fulfilling adult life, mentally, physically and emotionally. It is thus important to detect these children so that they can be given help in achieving this goal (Chang, 1987).

Prevalent among those unable to adjust to their experiences of childhood cancer was the worry of recurrence and second malignancies. This resulted in loss of orientation and prevented the patient making decisions about their future. Their purpose in life becomes distorted and here family therapy may result in positive steps towards gaining direction and self-esteem. Parental expectations are very important. If expectations of their child are high and they are treated as 'normal' then they will aspire to achieve, confidence increases and self-esteem can return.

Specific issues of physical or visible impairment, marriage, children and employment have been addressed to determine whether they resulted in maladjustment problems. Physical or visible impairments, such as amputation, scoliosis or sterility, were found to be coincidental in the psychological adjustment in these patients. That is patients who adjust well psychologically, do so regardless of any degree of impairment.

When marital status was examined, and many of their study group were over 21 years and of an age to marry, it was found that marriage amongst this group was lower than the national average. Of those who had married, their spouses were all aware of their partner's diagnosis prior to marriage and very few faltered over the decision with regard to potential fertility problems. Evaluating the influence of physical disability produced interesting results, which require further research. Women with visible disabilities were less likely to marry than men with visible disabilities. In fact, the more severe the disability the more likely the man was to marry.

Effects of cancer to offspring was a great concern. Many of these patients had produced healthy children. Li (1987) reports a study in which there were 8 cancer victims among 2328 offspring. The parents were, however, more health conscious and tended to take their children to the doctor more frequently.

Discrimination in employment was a problem for some of these survivors. In general the better adjusted the patient was to their previous cancer experience the more likely he was to be employed. Those who experienced discrimination were commonly given potential absenteeism as a reason, which was usually far from justifiable.

Difficulties regarding life insurance, mortgage conditions and entry in the police or military services are frequently due to misconceptions about life expectancy and late effects of treatment. Accurate factual information is required by the public and businesses.

As members of the health care team, it is essential to be able to identify those children who are experiencing psychological problems in order to provide appropriate support, which may involve individual and/or family counselling, education and support from more than one discipline.

Long-term follow-up

Koocher (1985) describes the importance of family assessment in order to detect any stresses which are unique to the family with a child who is a long-term survivor of cancer. These assessments need to be at regular intervals with adequate time given for families to discuss any issues which, if not addressed, may lead to psychosocial maladjustment. Fergusson et al. (1987) states that clinics for the follow-up of medical, emotional and learning needs of these children are very different from acute toxicities and life and death situation of newly diagnosed patients. However, these needs bring certain implications in terms of time and manpower.

Fergusson's report from the US Children's Cancer Study Group documented the time required to assess and evaluate potential late effects of these survivors. Examination of children who were not long-term survivors was approximately 37 minutes, whereas to assess potential problems in long-term survivors took 15 minutes longer. This examination/assessment did not include any additional time to address the family's need for support and information or referrals to other professional disciplines.

The implications for manpower requirements in the light of more children surviving their disease means that if each clinic visit takes approximately one hour, future out-patient clinics will have to develop separately from the 'acute toxicities clinic' with obvious implications on medical and nursing staff numbers.

There are children who experience childhood cancer who emerge as stronger individuals with a better sense of values, and the meaning of life becomes all the more important (Leightman and Friedman, 1975). As health professionals working with these children, our care can no longer be assessed only managing in terms of toxicities and survival rates but also on preparing these children and their families for the long-term psychosocial and physical sequelae of having lived with childhood cancer.

REFERENCES

Appleton, R.E., Farrell, K., Zaide, J. et al. (1990) Decline in head growth and cognitive impairment in survivors of acute lymphoblastic leukaemia. Archives of Disease in Childhood, 65(5), 530–534.

Aubier, F., Flamant, F., Brauner, R. et al. (1989) Male gonadal function after chemotherapy for solid tumors in childhood. Journal of Clinical Oncology, 7, 304–309.

Brown, I.H., Lee, T.J., Eden, O.B. et al. (1983) Growth and endocrine function after treatment for medulloblastoma. Archives of Disease in Childhood, 58, 722–727.

Chang, P. (1987) Personality characteristics and psychosocial adjustment of long-term survivors of childhood cancer. *Journal of Psychosomatic Oncology*, **5**, 43–47.

Clayton, P.E., Morris-Jones, P.H., Shalet, S.M. *et al.* (1988) Growth in children treated for acute lymphoblastic leukaemia. *Lancet*, **i**, 483–485.

Copeland, D.R., Dowell, R.E., Fletcher, J.B. *et al.* (1988) Neuropsychological effects of childhood cancer treatment. *Journal of Child Neurology*, **3**, 53–62.

de Vathaire, F., Schweisguth, O., Rodary, C. *et al.* (1989) Long-term risk of second malignant neoplasm after a cancer in childhood. *British Journal of Cancer*, **59**, 448–452.

Fergusson, J., Ruccione, K., Waskerwitz, M. *et al.* (1987) Time required to assess children for the late effects of treatment: A report from the Children's Cancer Study Group. *Cancer Nursing*, **10**(10), 300–310.

Gilberts, R. (1983) The evaluation of self-esteem. *Family Community Health*, **6**, 29–49.

Greenberg, H.S., Kazak, A.E. and Meadows, A.T. (1989) Psychologic functioning in 8 to 16 year old cancer survivors and their parents. *Journal of Pediatrics*, **114**, 488–493.

Ingram, I., Mott, M.G., Mann, J.R. *et al.* (1987) Second malignancies in children treated for non-Hodgkin's lymphoma and T cell leukaemia with the UKCCSG regimens. *British Journal of Cancer*, **55**, 463–466.

Jannoun, L. (1983) Are cognitive and educational development affected by age at which prophylactic therapy is given in acute lymphoblastic leukemia? *Archives of Disease in Childhood*, **58**, 953–958.

Kirk, J.A., Stevens, M.M., Menser, M.A. *et al.* (1987) Growth failure and growth-hormone deficiency after treatment for acute lymphoblastic leukaemia. *Lancet*, **ii**, 190–192.

Koocher, G. (1985) Psychosocial care of the child cured of cancer. *Paediatric Nursing*, **11**(2), 91–93.

Koocher, G. and O'Malley, J. (1981) *The Damocles Syndrome. Psychosocial Consequences of Surviving Childhood Cancer*, McGraw-Hill, New York.

Kreuser, E.D., Hetzel, W.D., Heit, W. *et al.* (1988) Reproductive and endocrine gonadal functions in adults following multidrug chemotherapy for acute lymphoblastic or undifferentiated leukaemia. *Journal of Clinical Oncology*, **6**, 588–595.

Kushner, B.H., Zauber, A. and Tan, C.T.C. (1988) Second malignancies after childhood Hodgkin's disease. The Memorial Sloan-Kettering Cancer Center experience. *Cancer*, **62**, 1364–1370.

Lannering, B. and Albertsson-Wiklund, K. (1987) Growth hormone release in children after cranial irradiation. *Hormone Research*, **27**, 13–22.

Lansky, S., List, M., Ritter-Sterr, C. *et al.* (1985) Late effects. Psychosocial. *Clinical Oncology*, **4**, 239–246.

Larcombe, I.J., Walker, J., Charleton, A. *et al.* (1990) Impact of childhood cancer on return to normal schooling. *British Medical Journal*, **301**, 169–171.

Leightman, S.R. and Friedman, S.B. (1975) Social and psychological development of adolescents and the relationship to chronic illness. *Medical Clinics of North America*, **59**, 1314–1328.

Leiper, A.D., Stanhope, R., Kitching, P. *et al.* (1987) Precocious and premature puberty associated with treatment of acute lymphoblastic leukaemia. *Archives of Disease in Childhood*, **62**, 1107–1112.

Li, F. (1987) Genetic studies of survivors of childhood cancer. *American Journal of Pediatric Haematology and Oncology*, **9**, 104–106.

Lipshultz, S.E., Colan, S.D., Gelber, R.D. *et al.* (1991) Late cardiac effects of doxorubicin therapy for acute lymphoblastic leukemia in childhood. *New England Journal of Medicine*, **324**, 808–815.

Meadows, A. and Hobbie, W. (1986) The medical consequences of cure. *Cancer*, **58**, 524–528.

Milner, R.D.G. (1986) Which children should have growth hormone therapy? *Lancet*, **i**, 483–485.

Moroff, S.V. and Fuks, J.Z. (1986) Thyroid cancer following radiotherapy for Hodgkin's disease: A case report and review of the literature. *Medical Pediatric Oncology*, **14**, 216–220.

Ochs, J.J., Parvey, L.S., Whitaker, J.N. *et al.* (1983) Serial cranial computed-tomography scans in children with leukemia given two different forms of central nervous system therapy. *Journal of Clinical Oncology*, **1**, 793–798.

Packer, R.J., Zimmerman, R.A. and Bilaniuk, L.T. (1986) Magnetic resonance imaging in the evaluation of treatment related CNS damage. *Cancer*, **58**, 635–640.

Perry, M.C. and Yarbro, J.W. (eds) (1984) *Toxicity of Chemotherapy*, Grune & Stratton, New York.

Pinkerton, C.R. (1992) Avoiding chemotherapy related late effects in children with curable tumours. *Archives of Disease in Childhood*, **67**, 1116–1119.

Probert, J.C., Parker, B.R. and Kaplan, H.K. (1973) Growth retardation in children after megavoltage irradiation of the spine. *Cancer*, **32**, 634–639.

Pui, C.-H., Ribeiro, R.C., Hancock, M.L. *et al.* (1991) Acute myeloid leukemia in children treated with epipodophyllotoxins for acute lymphoblastic leukemia. *New England Journal of Medicine*, **325**, 1682–1687.

Reasoner, R.W. (1983) Enhancement of self-esteem in children and adolescents. *Family Community Health*, **6**, 51–64.

Sanders, J.E., Pritchard, S., Mahoney, P. *et al.* (1986) Growth and development following marrow transplantation for leukaemia. *Blood*, **68**, 1129–1135.

Schimpff, S.C., Diggs, C.H., Wiswell, J.G. *et al.* (1980) Radiation-related thyroid dysfunction: Implications for the treatment of Hodgkin's disease. *Annals of Internal Medicine*, **92**, 91–98.

Speyer, J.L., Green, M.D., Kramer, E. *et al.* (1988) Protective effect of the bispiperazinedione ICRF-187 against doxorubicin induced cardiac toxicity in women with advanced breast cancer. *New England Journal of Medicine*, **319**, 745–752.

Tucker, M.A., Coleman, C.N., Cox, R.S. *et al.* (1988) Risk of second cancers after treatment for Hodgkin's disease. *New England Journal of Medicine*, **318**, 76–81.

Wallace, M., Reiter, P. and Pendergrass, T. (1987) Parents of long-term survivors of childhood cancer: A preliminary survey to characterize concerns and needs. *Oncology Nursing Forum*, **14**(3), 39–43.

Wallace, W.H.B., Shalet, S.M., Morris-Jones, P.H. *et al.* (1990) Effect of abdominal irradiation on growth in boys treated for a Wilms' tumour. *Medical Pediatric Oncology*, **18**, 441–446.

Wofford, L. (1987) 'Cured . . . What now?' *Paediatric Nursing*, **13**(4), 252–254.

Yeung, S.T., Yoong, C., Spink, J. *et al.* (1991) Functional myocardial impairment in children treated with anthracyclines for cancer. *Lancet*, **337**, 816–818.

Index